SIMPLY
REFLEXOLOGY

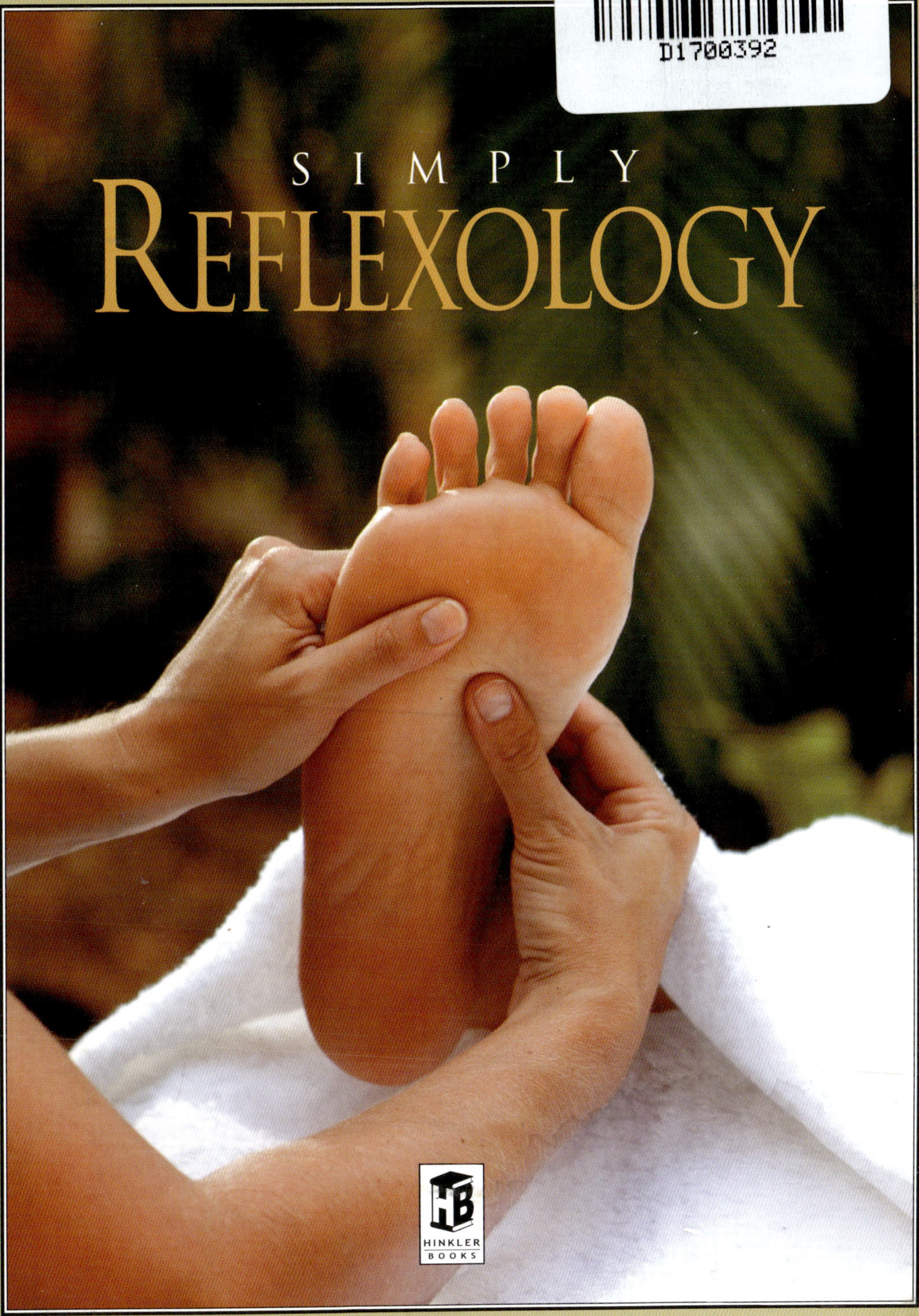

HB
HINKLER
BOOKS

Author: Claire Wynn
Art Director: Karen Moores
Editor: Jane Keighley and Hinkler Books Studio
Graphic Artist: Susie Allen
Photographer: Glenn Weiss
Model: Keft Burdell

First published in 2006
by Hinkler Books Pty Ltd
45–55 Fairchild Street
Heatherton Victoria 3202 Australia
www.hinklerbooks.com

Text © Claire Wynn 2006
Design © Hinkler Books Pty Ltd 2006

9 11 10
11 10

All rights reserved. No part of this publication may be reproduced, stored in a retrieval system, or transmitted in any way or by any means, electronic, mechanical, photocopying, recording, or otherwise, without the prior written permission of Hinkler Books Pty Ltd.

Printed and bound in China

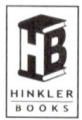

ISBN: 9 7817 4157 958 1

The publishers and their respective employees or agents will not accept responsibility for injury or damage occasioned to any person as a result of participation in the activities described in this book.

CONTENTS

WHAT IS REFLEXOLOGY? 5	UPPER ARCH 30
HISTORY OF REFLEXOLOGY 7	LOWER ARCH 32
BENEFITS OF REFLEXOLOGY 9	HEEL 34
GLOSSARY 10	INSIDE OF THE FEET 35
HOW TO USE THIS BOOK 11	OUTSIDE OF THE FEET 38
	TOP OF THE FEET 39
PREPARING FOR A SESSION . . . 13	INNER ARCH 40
WHAT YOU WILL NEED 13	FINISHING SEQUENCE 41
GETTING COMFORTABLE 13	WHOLE SEQUENCE 42
RECOMMENDATIONS 14	
HAND EXERCISES 14	HANDS 44
	ANATOMY OF THE HAND 44
BASIC TECHNIQUES 16	REFLEX POINTS OF THE HANDS . . . 45
BASIC THUMB WALKING	STARTING THE SESSION 46
TECHNIQUE 16	RELAXERS 46
HOOK IN AND UP METHOD 18	PALMS AND FRONT OF
KNUCKLES 18	THE FINGERS 49
	BACK OF THE HANDS AND FINGERS . 52
FEET 19	
ANATOMY OF THE FOOT 19	FACE AND EARS 54
REFLEX POINTS OF THE FEET 20	REFLEX POINTS OF THE
STARTING THE SESSION 22	FACE AND EARS 54
RELAXERS 22	STARTING THE SESSION 56
BIG TOE 25	FACE 57
REST OF THE TOES 27	EAR 62
BALLS OF THE FEET 28	ABOUT THE AUTHOR 64

5 4 3 2 1
1 2 3 4 5
1
2
3
4
5
1
2
3
4
5

The 10 energy zones of the body
5 4 3 2 1
1 2 3 4 5
Midline

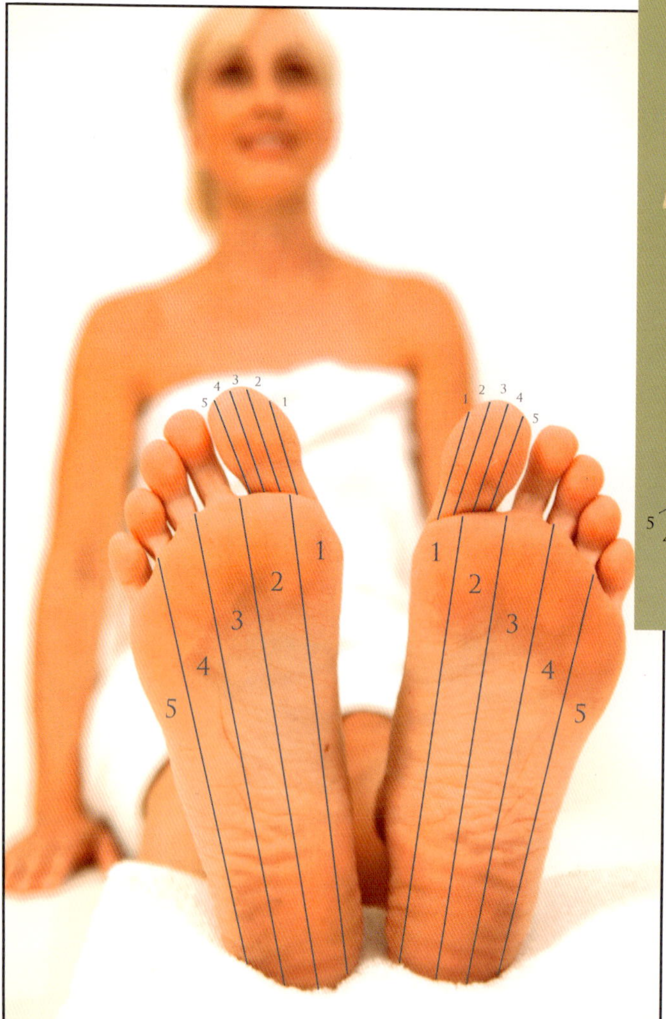

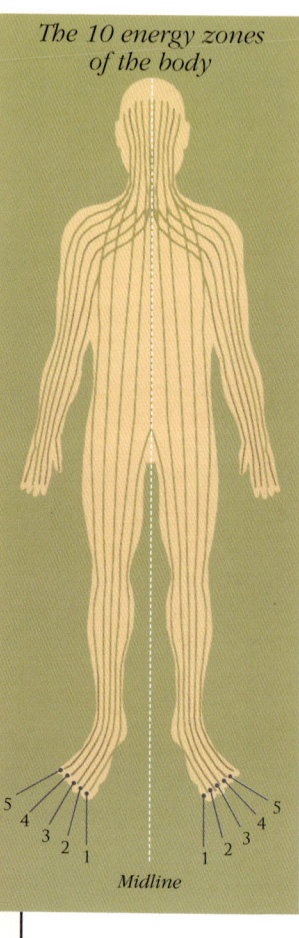

What is Reflexology?

Reflexology is a science based on the principle that there are reflexes in the feet, hands and face that directly correspond with glands, organs and parts of the body. **Better Health with Foot Reflexology**

Reflexology is a unique method of using the thumb and fingers to stimulate reflex areas that relate to different parts of the body.

Working on these reflexes can trigger physiological changes that empower the body and mind to heal itself.

Reflexology works on many levels. It is a deeply relaxing therapy that stimulates the circulatory and lymphatic systems. It also helps to release any blockages in the flow of energy around the body and allows energy to move freely, enabling us to stay healthy.

The body is divided from head to toe into 10 energy zones. There are five zones on each side of the midline, which runs down the centre of the body. Energy is constantly flowing through these zones. The flow of energy terminates in the feet and hands, forming reflex points.

The right foot represents the right side of the body and the left foot represents the left side of the body. Where there are organs on both sides of the body, for example the lungs, the right lung will be found on the right foot and the left lung on the left foot.

Reflexology is a holistic therapy where the whole body is always treated. As each gland and organ is interconnected, stimulation will lead to improved health and a total sense of wellbeing.

Simply Reflexology is an introduction to the methods and techniques of reflexology. To experience the full benefits of reflexology, book a session with a qualified reflexologist. I hope you enjoy practising and receiving the techniques outlined in this book.

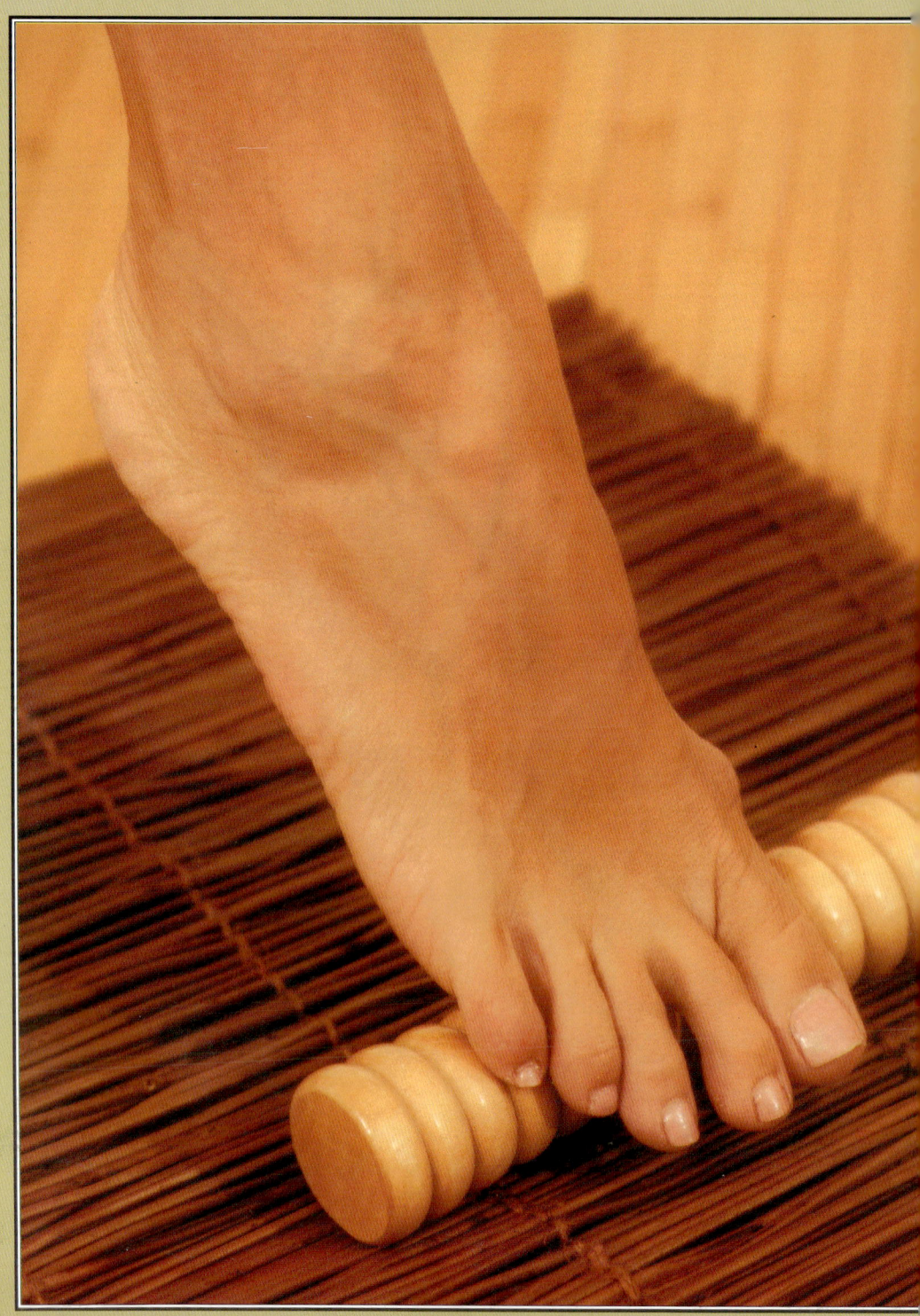

History of Reflexology

Reflexology has its foundations in both the old world and the new. Illustrations from ancient texts in China, Japan, Russia and Egypt show that these civilisations worked on the feet to promote good health. It is thought that in China the early physicians made equal use of acupressure and reflexology. However, as they further developed acupressure and acupuncture, reflexology became forgotten. Today, many of the same ancient techniques have been rediscovered, researched and developed into modern reflexology.

In 1917 Dr William H. Fitzgerald laid the foundations of modern reflexology with his theory of 'Zone Therapy'. Dr Fitzgerald had discovered, through experimentation and case studies, that he could relieve pain in other parts of the body by working the corresponding 'zone' in the feet or hands.

Inspired by his work, American physiotherapist Eunice Ingam further developed his theory through more painstaking research and discovered that the feet were more responsive to pressure than the hands. She also discovered that the zone theory could be extended, and she reproduced a map of the body onto the feet with the corresponding reflexes that affect each organ, gland and part of the body.

The first Reflexology Association was set up in America in 1973 and since then reflexology associations have been formed around the world. This has allowed the practice of reflexology to develop and grow through education and research and it is now one of the leading forms of complementary therapies. Reflexology has been used in many aged and palliative care facilities to improve the quality of care for in-patients.

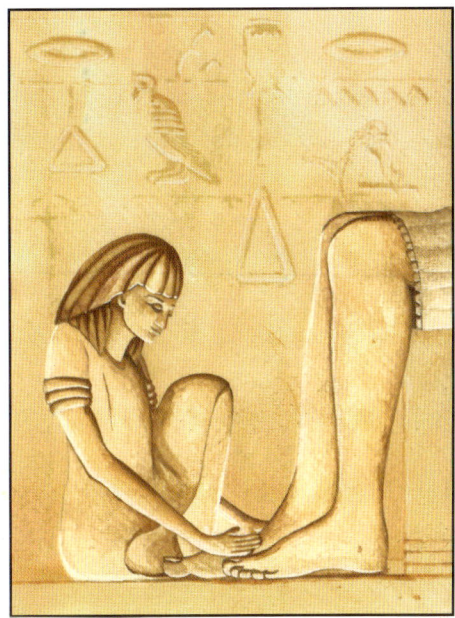

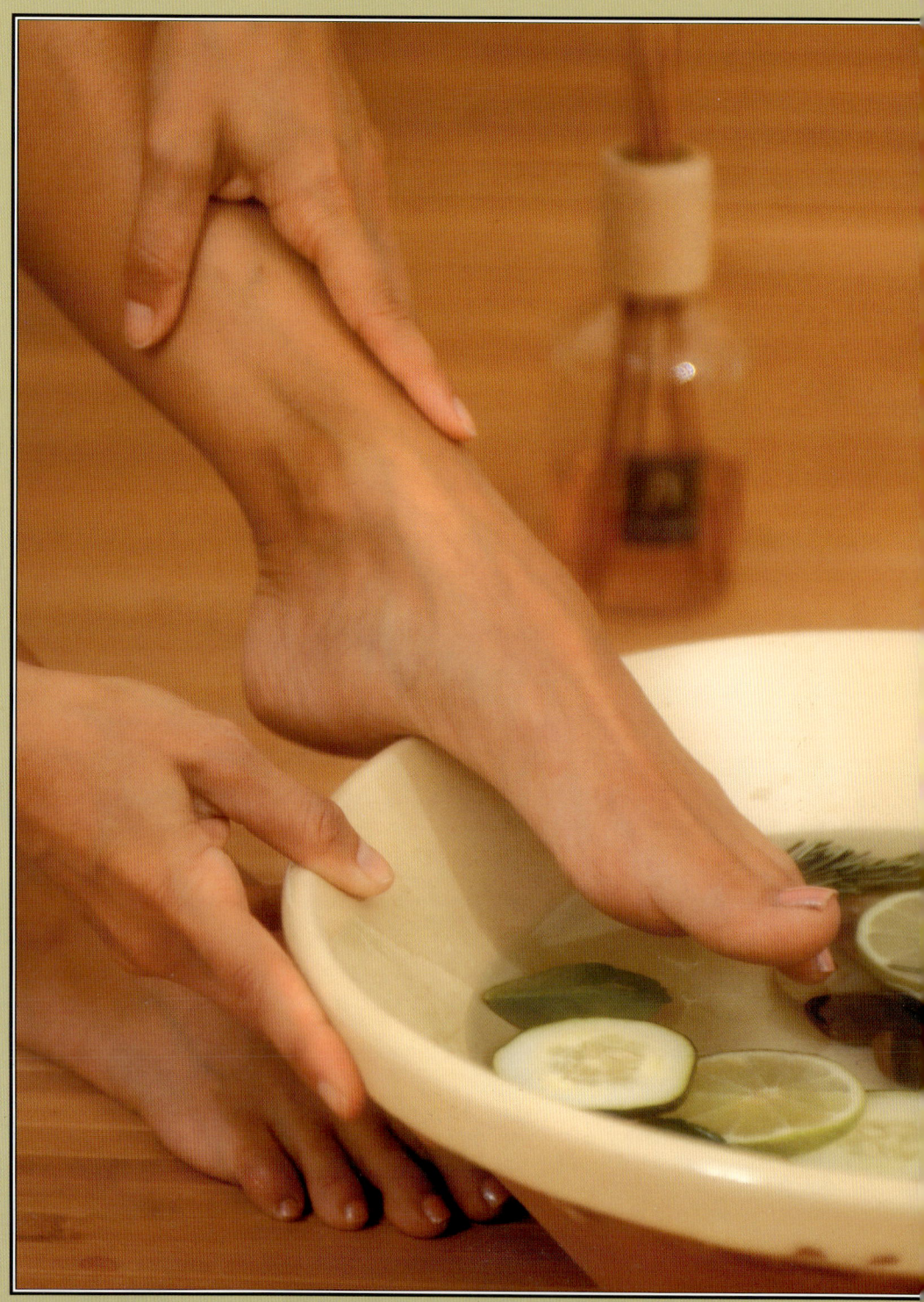

Benefits of Reflexology

Reflexology helps to harmonise your body. It can have a positive effect on your health in many ways and is suitable for people of all ages. It is a powerful preventative therapy and also promotes a deep sense of relaxation.

Reflexology clears away blockages in the flow of energy around the body, which helps to:

- Reduce stress and tension
- Improve circulation
- Alleviate pain
- Balance the nervous system
- Boost the lymphatic function
- Stimulate a sluggish and congested system
- Improve sleeping patterns
- Increase energy and vitality
- Detoxify and cleanse the body
- Improve skin tone and condition
- Promote self-healing

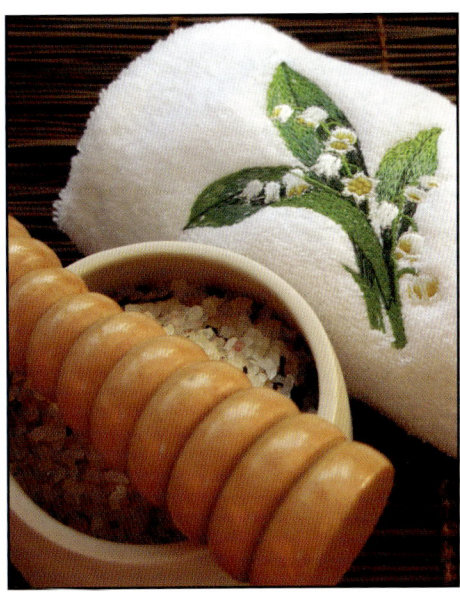

Glossary

Dorsal
Relating to the back surface.

Lateral
Towards the outside edges of the body.

Medial
Towards the centre of the body.

Palmar
Relating to the palm of the hand.

Plantar
Relating to the sole of the foot.

Reflex
A point or area on the feet, hands, face or ears that relates to a gland, organ or part of the body.

Thumb Walking or Caterpillar Walking
The basic technique used in reflexology (refer to page 16, Basic Thumb Walking Technique).

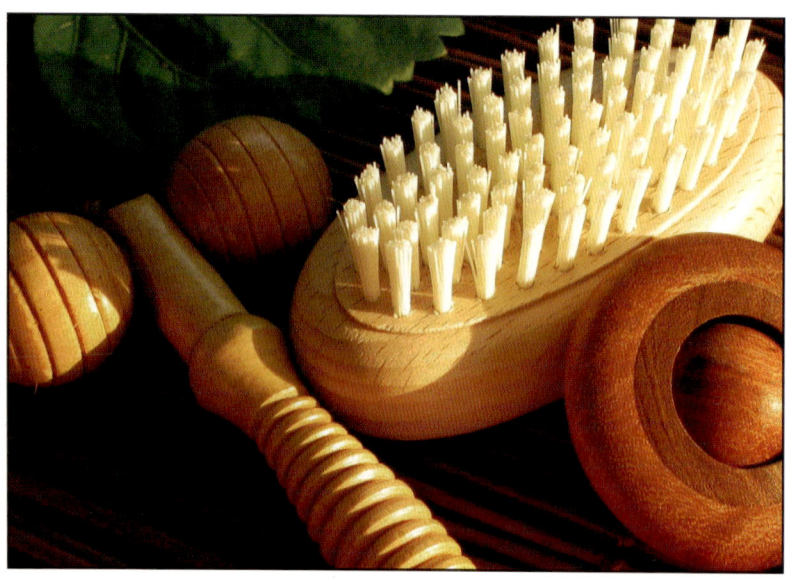

How to Use This Book

While many reflexes are the same on both feet, there are some differences between the left and the right foot. When treating the feet, it is important to begin with the right foot. Complete all reflexes on the right foot, then move on to the left foot in the same manner, before performing the final sequence.

Symbols have been used throughout this book to indicate which foot each treatment is performed on. Most sequences will be performed on both feet, but there are a number that are only done on the right foot and corresponding ones that are only done on the left foot.

As you proceed through the sequence, refer to the symbols below to see which sequence is performed on which foot.

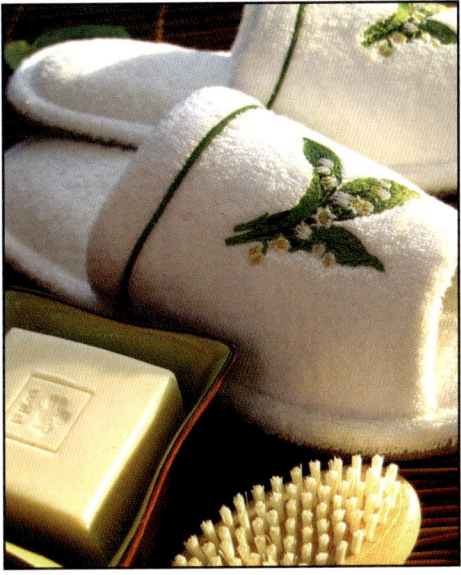

B Both feet

R Right foot only

L Left foot only

Begin with the right foot, carrying out in order all the reflexes marked **B** or **R**. Complete all the reflexes except for the solar plexus hold on the right foot, and then return to the start of the foot section to work on the left foot. Again, work through the series of reflexes in order, this time carrying out all reflexes marked **B** or **L**. Finish the sequence with the solar plexus hold.

To see a summary of the entire foot sequence in order, refer to pages 42–3. Note, there is no difference between the reflex points of the hands. When using the hand section of the book, the same sequence can be performed on both hands.

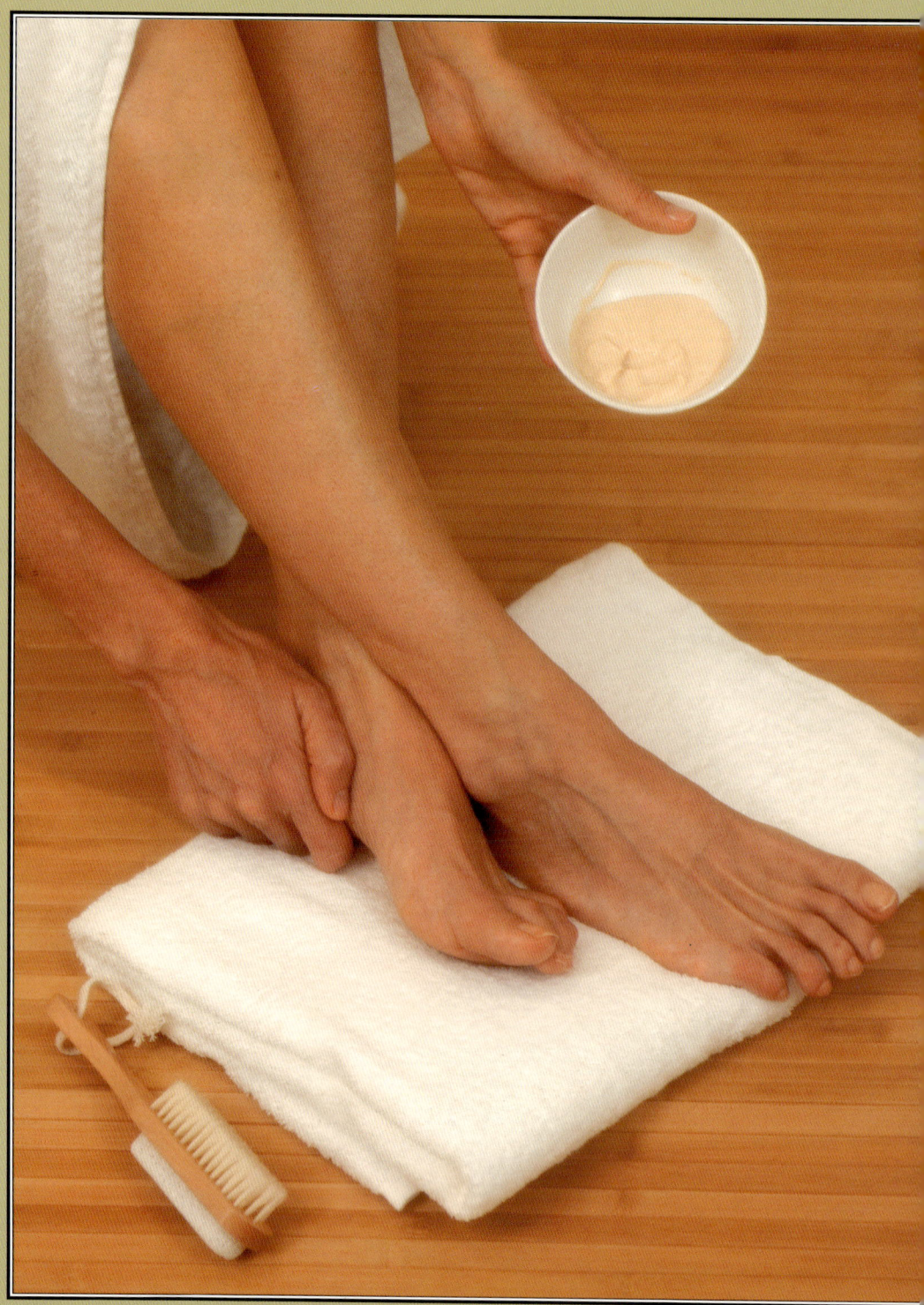

Preparing for a Session

What You Will Need

- Hand or foot cream
- Towels (one for yourself and one to keep your partner's feet warm)

It is important not to use too much cream, as your thumbs may slip. If you have applied too much, wipe it off with your towel.

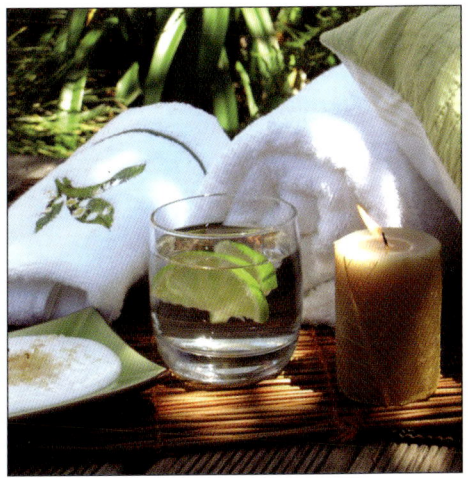

Getting Comfortable

Make sure your partner is comfortable:

- Use a massage table or reclining chair
- Ensure the room is at a comfortable temperature – have a blanket or towel on hand
- Have pillows available to support the head and to place under the legs to support the lower back if necessary.

Make sure you are comfortable:

- Use a comfortable stool or chair at an appropriate height to your partner, so you are not stooping – a gas-lift stool is ideal
- Wear comfortable clothes that allow for an easy range of movement
- Ensure everything you need is within reach and you are able to access both feet easily
- Ensure your nails are trimmed short.

Simply Reflexology · 13

Recommendations

There are very few occasions when you can't use reflexology as it is a gentle therapy. However it is recommended:

- Not to treat women in the first trimester of pregnancy
- To ask your partner to seek their doctor's advice if they are undergoing chemotherapy or any intensive medical treatment
- To always use gentle pressure and short sessions when working with the elderly or infirm
- Never to treat an area with broken skin or inflammation
- To treat babies for only five minutes using gentle stroking
- To treat diabetics for a shorter time as they may have thinner skin and bruise easily

If you can't work on the foot, you can always work the corresponding hand. If you have any concerns, always seek professional advice.

Hand Exercises

To provide a fuller range of movement and prevent injury, it is important to loosen your hands before commencing reflexology treatment.

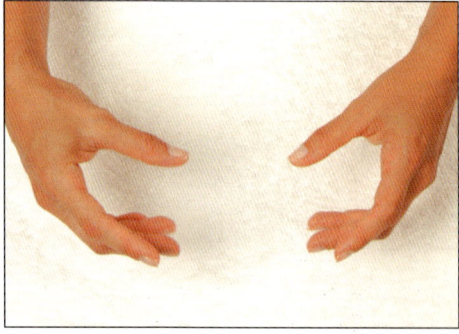

Loosely shake out both hands.

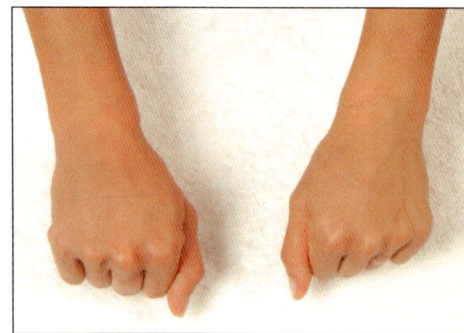

Make a fist with both hands. Squeeze tightly for 3–5 seconds and release. Relax your hands for a few seconds, then repeat the sequence 3 times.

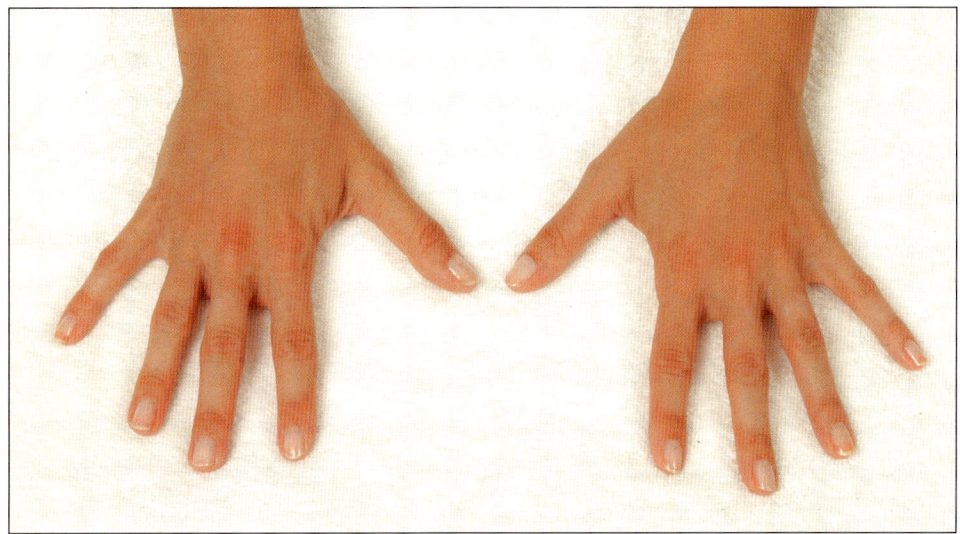

Spread the fingers of both hands wide, stretching them as far as you can. Hold this position for 3–5 seconds and release. Relax your hands for a few seconds, then repeat the sequence 3 times.

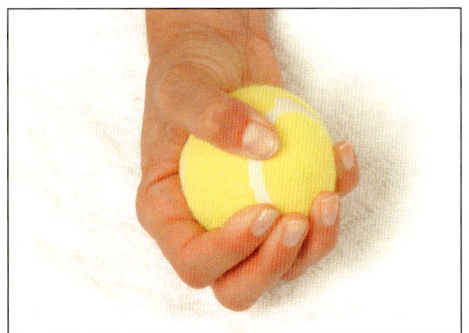

Hold a squash, tennis or stress ball and squeeze it tightly in your hand for 3–5 seconds. Relax your hand for a few seconds, then repeat the sequence 3 times. Place the ball in your other hand and repeat.

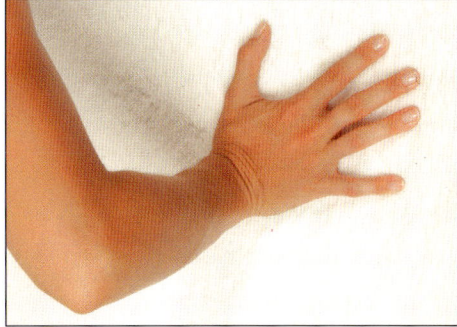

Place the palm of one hand flat against the wall and straighten your arm. Lean slightly into the wall, so that your weight is being supported by your palm. Hold for 3–5 seconds, release and repeat 3 more times. Swap hands and repeat the sequence.

Basic Techniques

There are three main techniques used in reflexology: basic thumb walking (or caterpillar walking), the hook in and up method, and using the knuckles.

Basic Thumb Walking Technique

Thumb walking is the main technique used in reflexology and you will be amazed how effective it is. I also like to think of it as 'caterpillar walking' and, if you can imagine how a caterpillar moves along a branch, you'll see there is a great similarity.

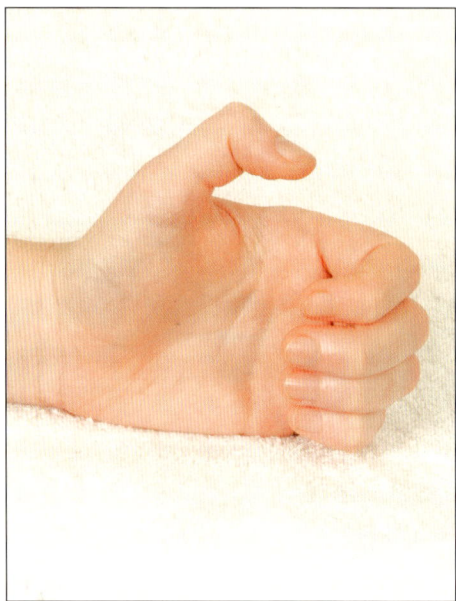
Bending the thumb

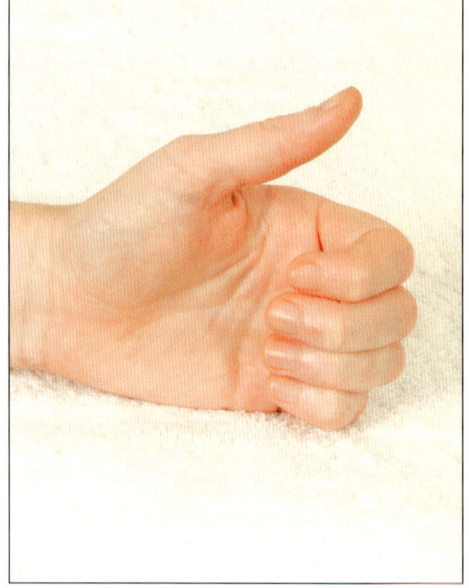
Straightening the thumb

Just bend your thumb and then straighten it. As you repeat this motion, move your thumb along in small steps. The smaller the movement, the greater the coverage you will get in the area you are working on.

It may feel awkward at first but it will soon feel natural, and if you are practising on your free hand you will start to feel the improvements in your technique. Working on yourself is also a great way to assess and modify your pressure.

While practising, notice the difference between using the flat of your thumb and using the side. You will be able to exert more pressure using the side of your thumb. You will also notice the importance of keeping your nails trimmed short.

You can also perform the caterpillar movement with other fingers.

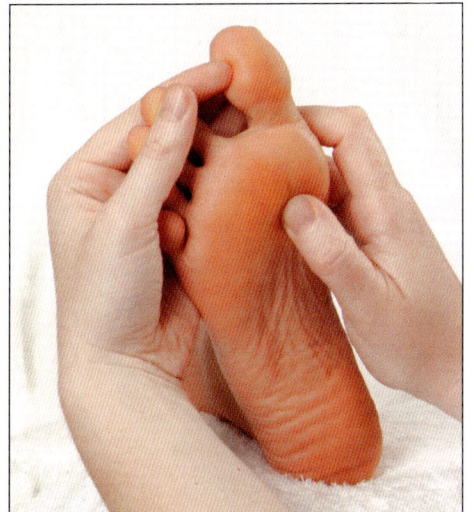

Flat of the thumb

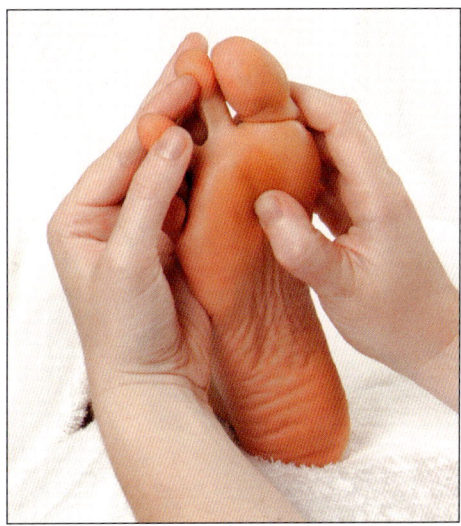

Side of the thumb

Practising the thumb walking technique

It's best to practise, practise, practise this technique!

- Practise the technique on yourself. Try it on different parts of your body, such as your arm, your free hand, or, if you are flexible enough, your own feet.

- You can also practise the technique on a tennis ball. Try practising using a ball while you're sitting on a train or bus.

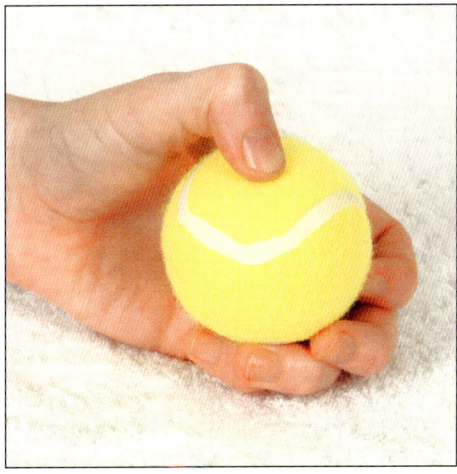

SIMPLY REFLEXOLOGY · 17

Hook In and Up Method

Locate the desired reflex and place your thumb vertically on top of it. Press down, hook your thumb in and pull it up.

This method really gets deeply into the reflexes and is used particularly on the pituitary gland. Be careful though, as it can be quite painful.

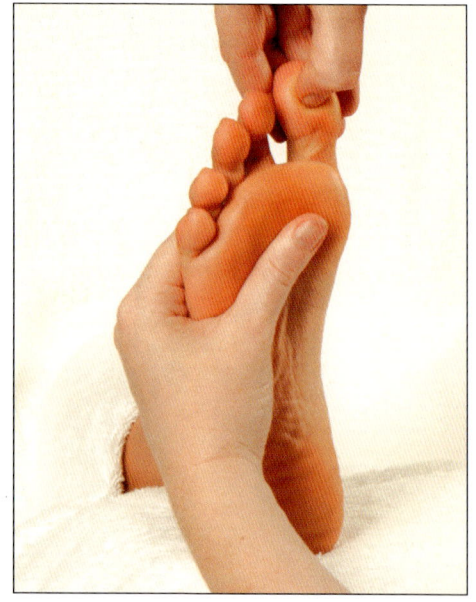

Knuckles

Bend your fingers and drag the index finger knuckle in a sweeping motion over the relevant area, pressing down as you move across the foot. Be careful when you use this technique, as you can exert more pressure on the foot than you realise.

This is a useful technique if you are working on someone with very thick skin on their feet or you need to work the balls of the feet and the heels. It is also a helpful technique to use if your thumbs are getting tired and sore during a session.

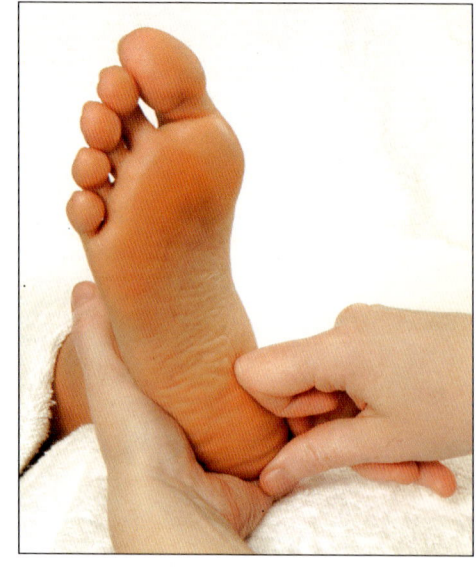

Feet

Anatomy of the Foot

Each foot is made up of 26 bones as well as muscles, ligaments and nerves.

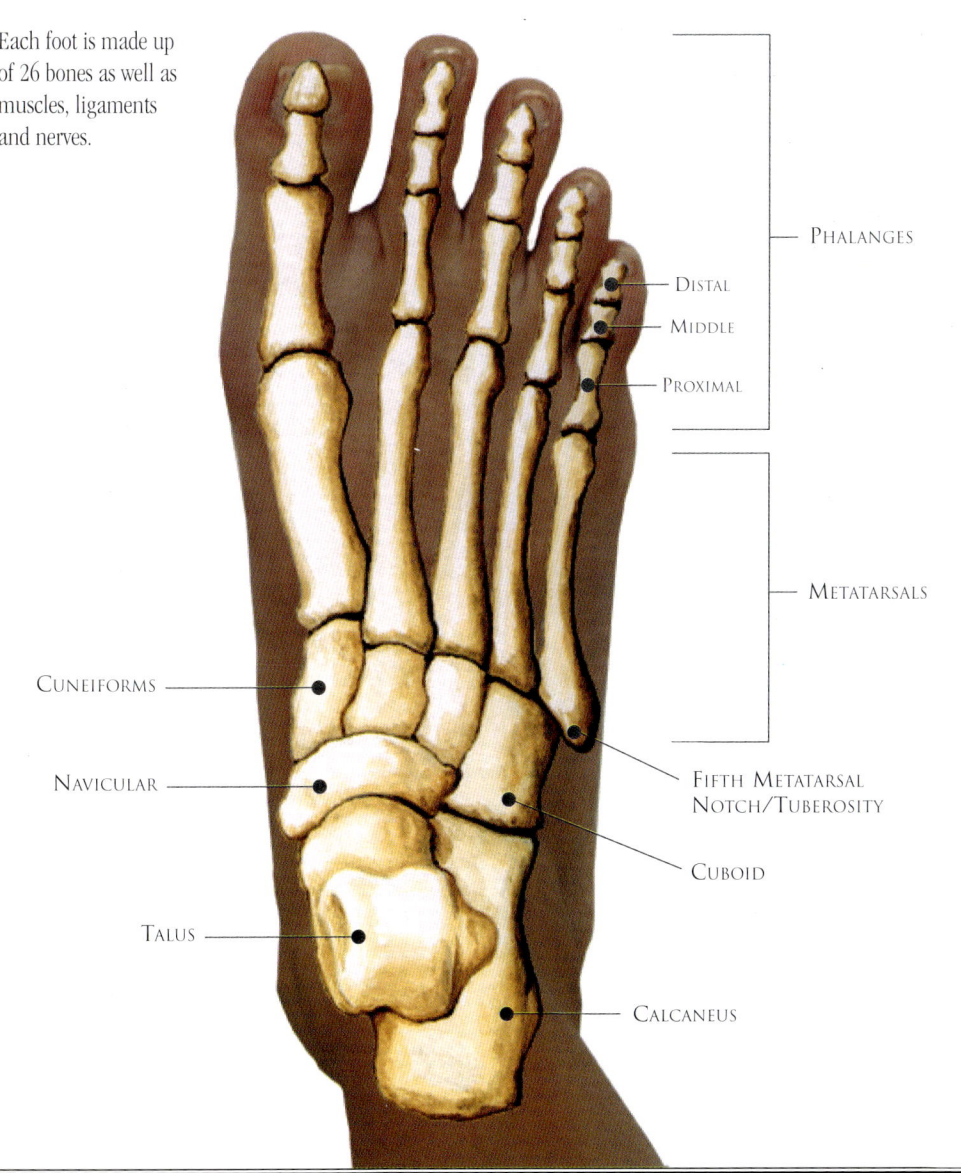

- Phalanges
  - Distal
  - Middle
  - Proximal
- Metatarsals
- Cuneiforms
- Navicular
- Fifth Metatarsal Notch/Tuberosity
- Cuboid
- Talus
- Calcaneus

Reflex Points of the Feet

Soles of the Feet (Plantar Aspect)

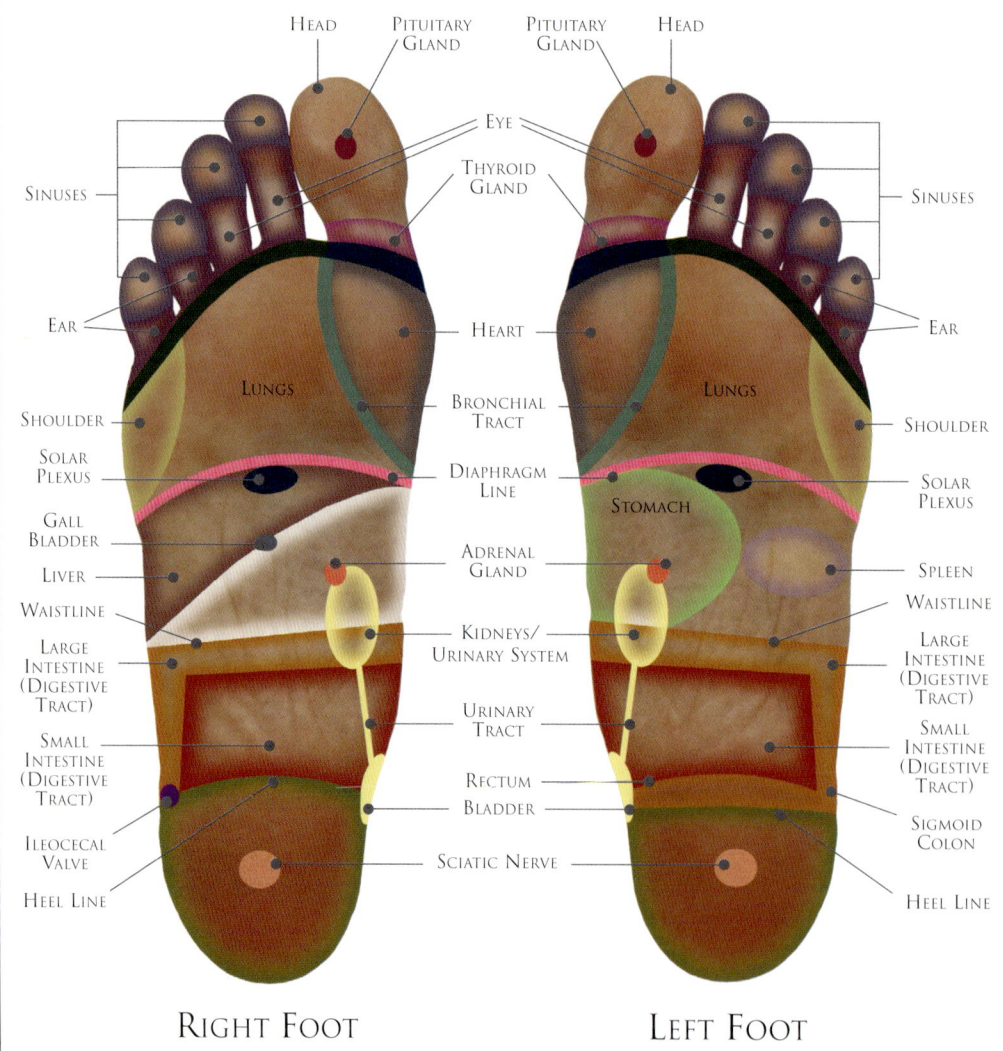

Inside of the Feet (Medial Aspect)

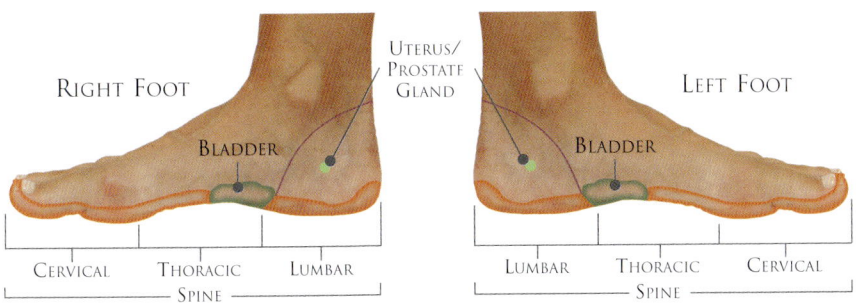

Outside of the Feet (Lateral Aspect)

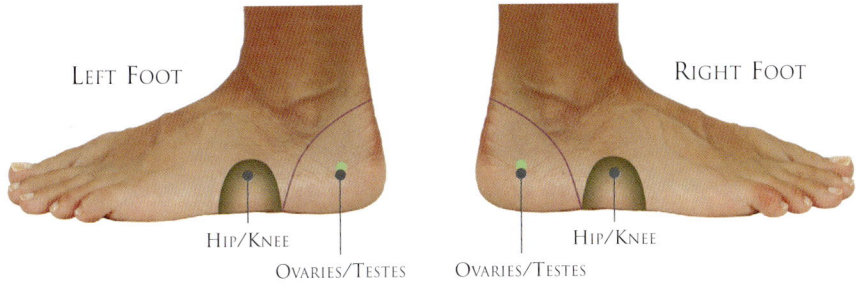

Top of the Feet (Dorsal Aspect)

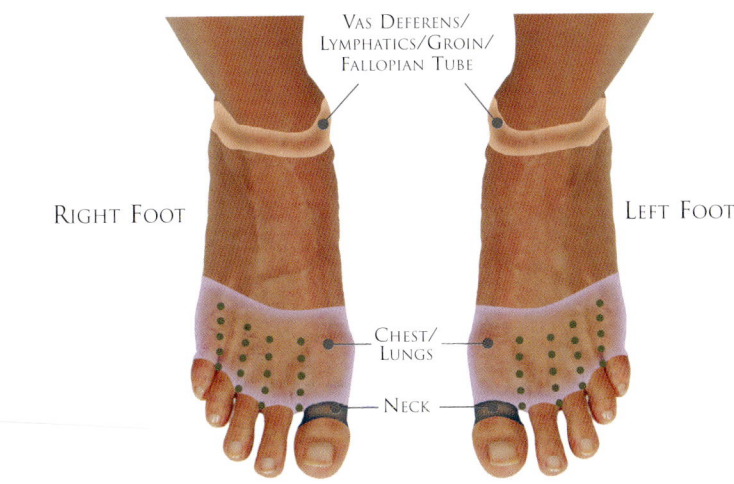

Starting the Session

Start the session by touching your partner's feet. Cup the feet with your hands. Remember it is important to begin with the right foot. Complete all appropriate reflexes on the right foot, then move onto the left foot in the same manner, before finishing with the solar plexus hold. Before commencing the session, apply cream to the feet.

Relaxers

Relaxers help reduce muscular tension in the feet, loosening them up and making them easier to work with. If your partner becomes tense, you can return to these exercises throughout the session.

Ankle Boogie B

Place the palms of your hands on either side of the ankle bone and gently move your hands from side to side. Perform this sequence for around 10–15 seconds.

Side to Side B

Cup the ball of the foot with both hands and gently move your hands from side to side. Perform this sequence for around 10–15 seconds.

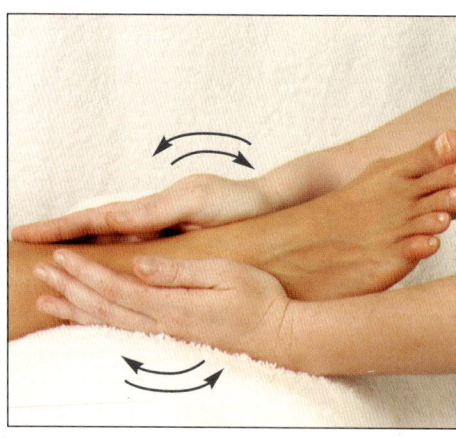

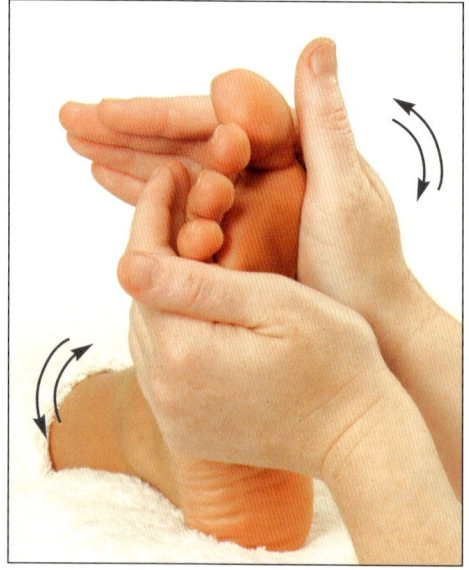

Metatarsal Kneading B

Place your fist into the ball of your partner's foot. At the same time, cup the dorsal aspect of the foot with your other hand. Push into the ball of the foot with your fist, while supporting with your other hand. Push in for three seconds and release. Repeat this sequence 3 times.

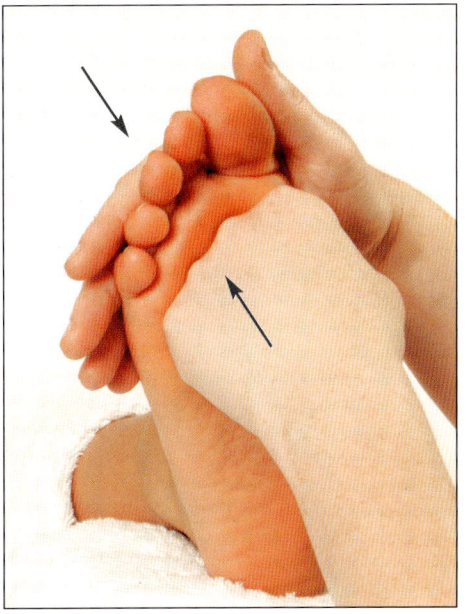

Lower Leg Massage B

Support your partner's foot with your holding hand. With your main hand, massage your partner's calf just above the ankle using a kneading motion. Perform this massage for a few seconds and then move up the leg, repeating the kneading technique. Continue until the entire calf up to the knee has been covered.

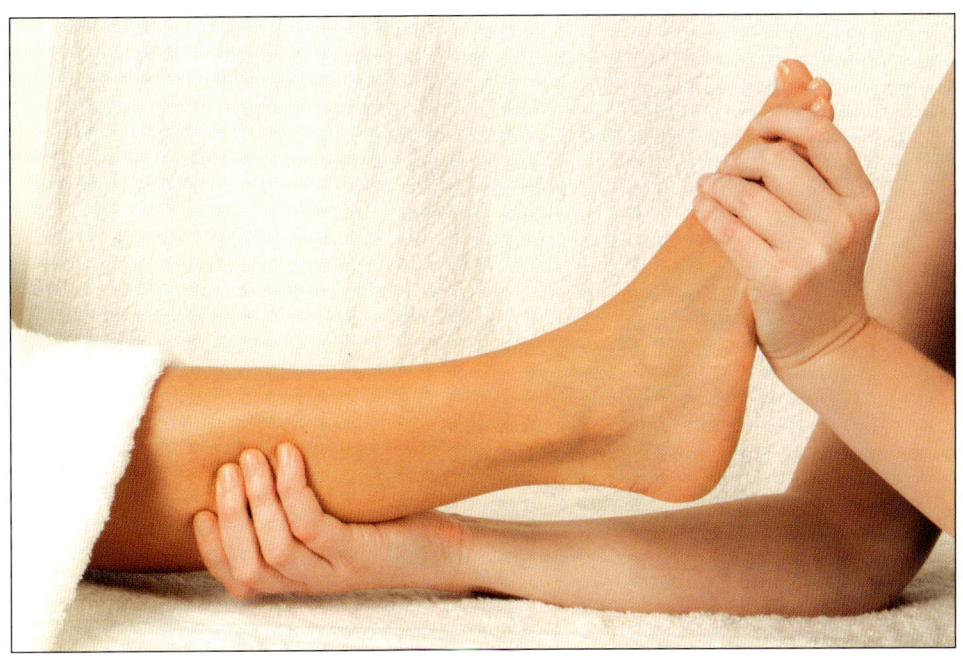

Relaxers *(continued)*

Diaphragm Relaxer B

Relaxing the diaphragm is excellent for relieving tension in the body and it also aids breathing.

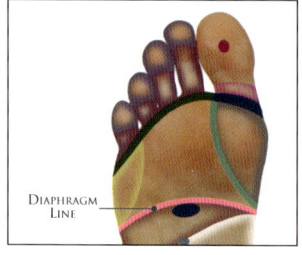

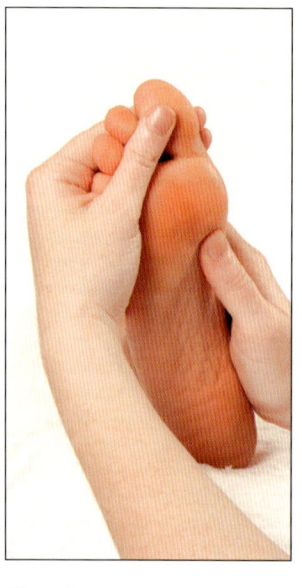

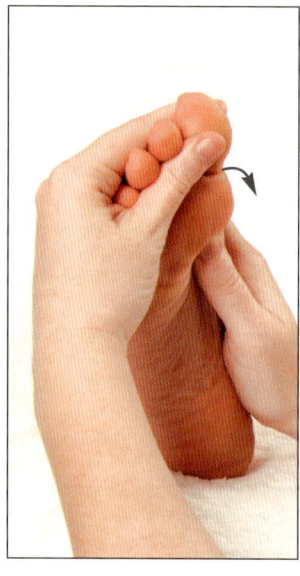

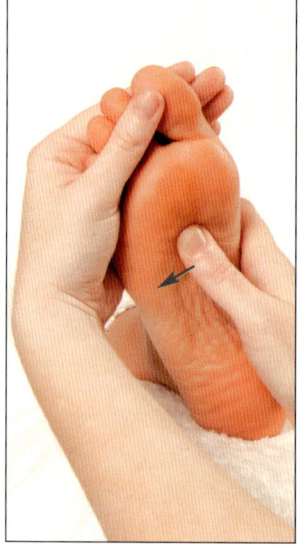

Step 1

Hold the right foot with your holding hand, fingers supporting the dorsal aspect of the foot.

Place the thumb of your main hand at the beginning of the diaphragm line under the big toe.

Step 2

Lift the foot over your thumb, using an up and over motion. Then lift the foot back off the thumb.

Step 3

Move your thumb slightly along the diaphragm line and repeat step 2. Repeat this sequence in small, gentle movements, covering the whole diaphragm line.

Change hands and repeat the sequence going back the other way along the diaphragm line.

Big Toe

The big toe encompasses the head, thyroid gland, neck and pituitary gland reflexes. Reflexology on the big toe will help with migraines and headaches, and sinus, ear, eye, neck, throat, jaw and facial problems.

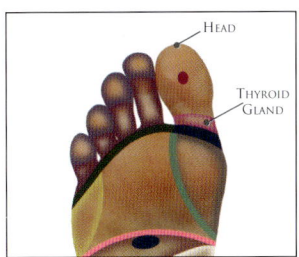

Head Reflex ⓑ

Hold the right foot in your left hand, supporting the toes with your left hand and working with your right hand. This is a good time to ask for feedback from your partner and to check that you are using a comfortable pressure on their feet.

Use your thumb to caterpillar vertically down the big toe in rows, starting at the top and moving to the neck of the toe. Cover the fleshy part of the big toe. Repeat 3 times.

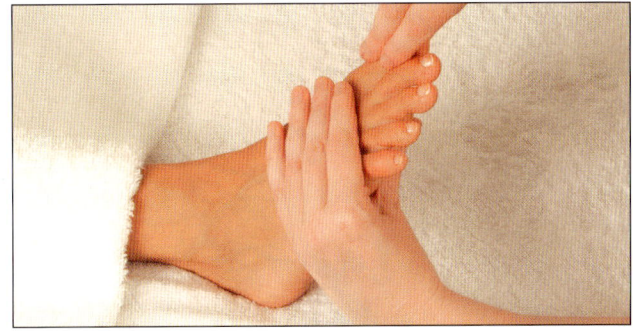

Holding the foot to perform the head reflex

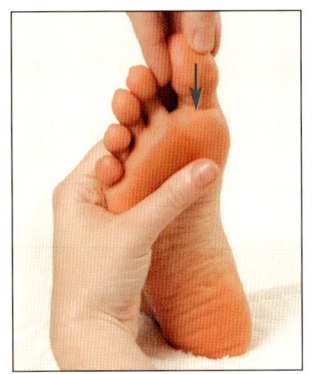

Caterpillaring down the head reflex

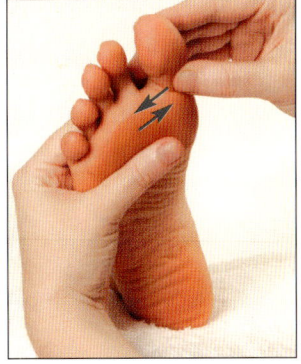

Thyroid Gland Reflex ⓑ

Caterpillar across the neck of the big toe horizontally towards the lateral side (outside) of the foot. Swap hands and repeat, working towards the medial side (inside) of the foot. Repeat 3 times.

SIMPLY REFLEXOLOGY · 25

Big Toe
(continued)

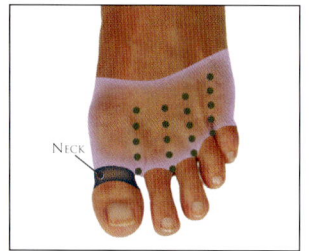
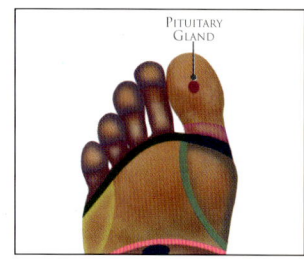

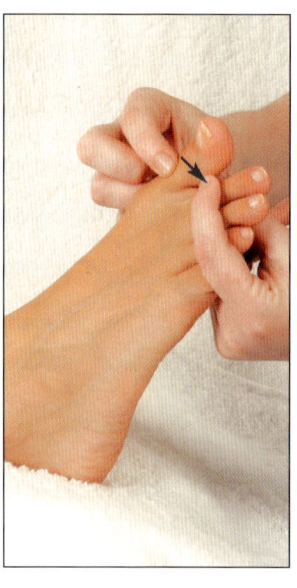
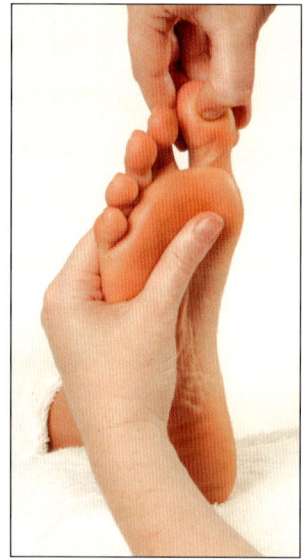
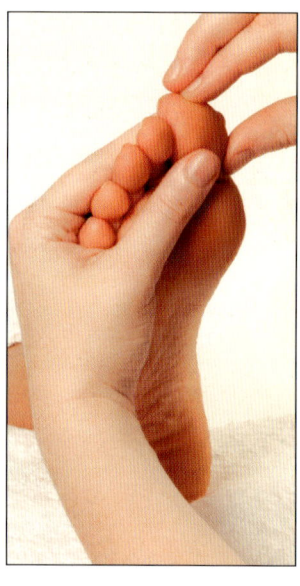

Neck Reflex

Using the index finger, caterpillar across the dorsal aspect of the big toe horizontally, working from the inside (or medial side) of the foot to the outside (or lateral side). Cover the whole toe. Repeat 3 times.

Pituitary Gland Reflex

Locate the pituitary gland reflex – this is in the centre of the footprint swirl on the big toe.

Use the hook in and up movement on the reflex. Repeat 3 times.

Head of the Toe

Place your middle finger on top of your index finger. Press both your fingers down gently on the tip of the big toe and massage it using a small rocking motion. Make sure you cover the whole head of the toe area.

Rest of the Toes

Reflexology on the remaining toes will help relieve sinusitis, allergies and hayfever, and teeth, gum, eye, hearing and balance problems.

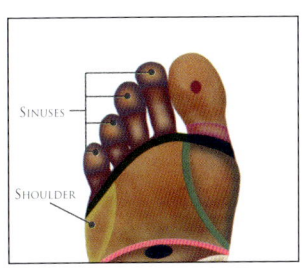

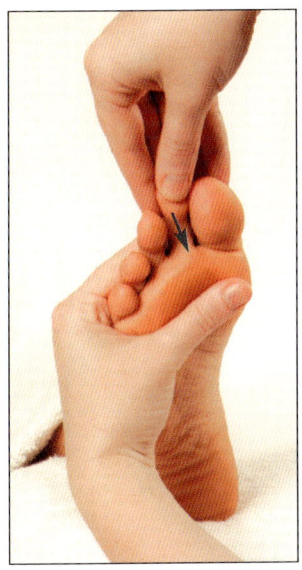

Front of the toe

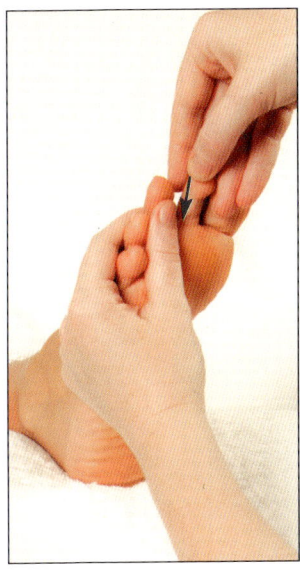

Side of the toe

Sinus Reflex

Support the toes with your holding hand. Caterpillar down the front of the second toe and then down one side. Work your way across the toes, repeating this sequence on each toe.

After completing the little toe, swap your holding hand and caterpillar back the other way across the foot, down the front and then down the other side of the toes. Repeat 3 times.

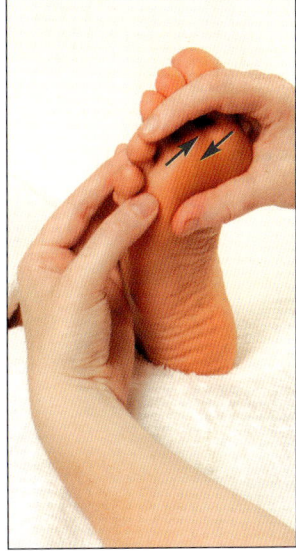

Shoulder Reflex

Caterpillar your thumb across the foot under the base of the toes, working first from lateral to medial side and then from medial to lateral. If you need more pressure, you can caterpillar with the side of your thumbs. Repeat 3 times each way. Swap your holding hand as you change directions.

SIMPLY REFLEXOLOGY · 27

Balls of the Feet

Stimulation of the reflex points on the balls of the feet helps with asthma and breathing difficulties, bronchitis and bronchial infections, and other lung conditions. It can also assist in boosting the immune system and help with menopause symptoms, dry skin and weight gain.

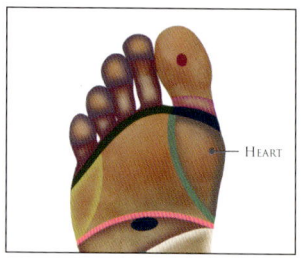

Heart Reflex B

Hold the foot with one hand supporting the toes and work with your main hand. Caterpillar over the entire heart reflex, first working horizontally over the whole area, then vertically and finally diagonally. Repeat the sequence 3 times.

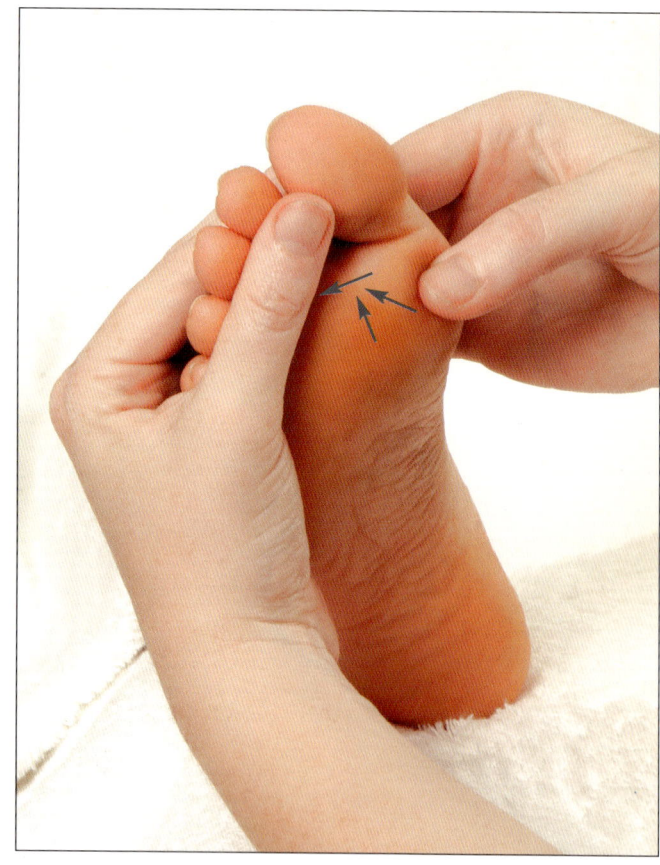

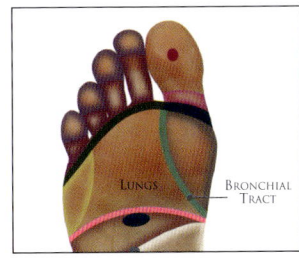

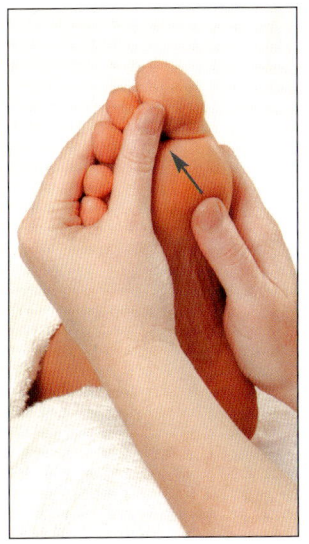

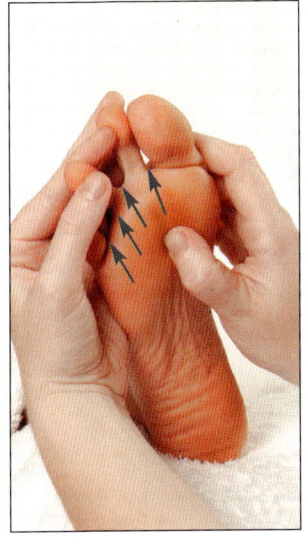

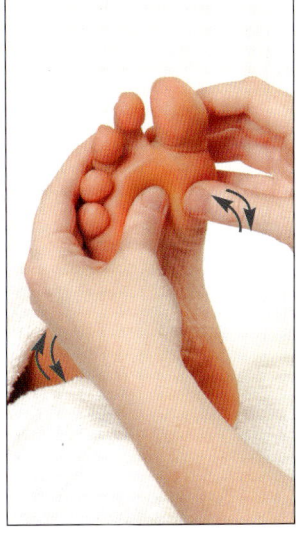

Bronchial Tract Reflex B

Caterpillar up the bronchial tract reflex, in between the big toe and second toe metatarsals, up towards the base of the toes. You can use the side of the thumb if necessary. Repeat 3 times.

Lung Reflex B

Caterpillar up between each metatarsal, working from between the first and second metatarsals to the fourth and fifth, and back again. Repeat 3 times each way. Swap your holding hand as you change directions. If necessary, hold the toes apart with your holding hand. This opens up the spaces between the metatarsals.

Metatarsal Wiggling B

Hold the foot with both hands, grasping below the base of the little toe on the metatarsal with one hand and below the base of the fourth toe on the metatarsal with the other. Gently wiggle your hands back and forth five or six times. Move up the foot repeating this sequence on each pair of metatarsals until you reach the big toe. Repeat the sequence moving back down the foot until you reach the little toe.

SIMPLY REFLEXOLOGY · 29

Upper Arch

Working on the upper arch area will help heal and prevent digestive and stomach problems, diabetes, hypoglycaemia, liver and gall bladder conditions, nervous disorders, fatigue, inflammatory conditions and adrenal gland problems.

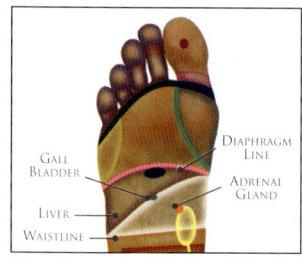

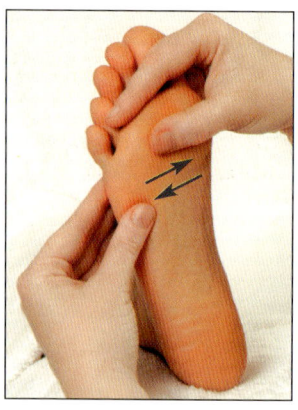
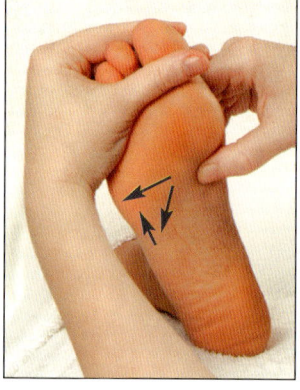
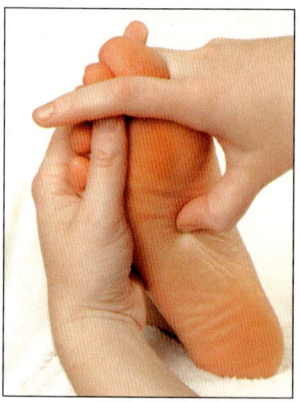

Diaphragm Line B

When working on the left foot, perform this sequence before moving on to the stomach and spleen.

Caterpillar horizontally along the diaphragm line, working one way with one thumb and back with the other. Repeat 3 times each way.

Liver Reflex R

Caterpillar over the triangular liver reflex area horizontally, then vertically and finally diagonally, ensuring the whole reflex is covered. Repeat 3 times.

Gall Bladder Reflex R

Locate the gall bladder, which is halfway along the diagonal line of the liver reflex. Use your thumb to hook in and up. Repeat 3 times.

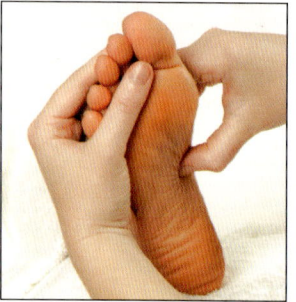

Adrenal Gland Reflex B

When working on the left foot, perform the stomach and spleen reflex before doing the adrenal gland reflex.

Locate the adrenal reflex by first locating the waistline. Follow it to the medial (or inside) edge, measure one thumb's width up towards the diaphragm line and use your thumb to hook in and up. Repeat 3 times.

Be very careful of the tendon, as this can be painful when pushed on. To locate it, gently bend the toes back. You should see the tendon clearly.

30 · SIMPLY REFLEXOLOGY

Stomach and Spleen Reflexes L

Complete the diaphragm line sequence (see page 30) on the left foot before moving on to the stomach and spleen.

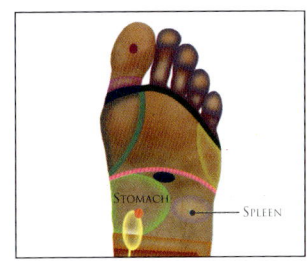

Starting at the inside (or medial side) of the foot, caterpillar with your thumb over the stomach reflex horizontally 3 times. Swap your holding hand and caterpillar horizontally 3 times across the spleen reflex, starting from the outside (or lateral side) of the foot.

Each time swapping hands, caterpillar 3 times vertically over the stomach reflex and then over the spleen reflex. Finish by caterpillaring diagonally 3 times over the stomach reflex and the spleen reflex. Make sure you have covered the whole area of both reflexes.

Once you've completed the stomach and spleen, move on to the adrenal gland sequence on page 30.

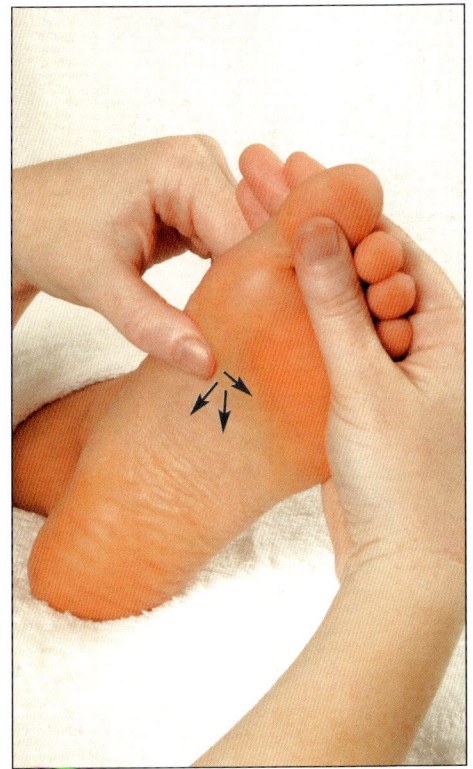

Stomach reflex

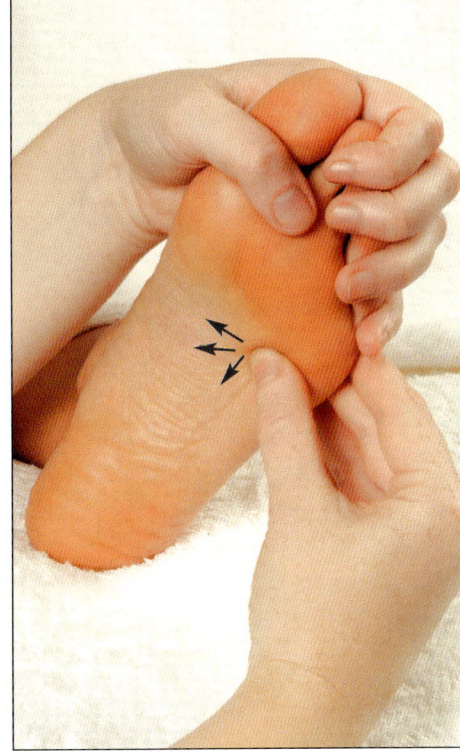

Spleen reflex

SIMPLY REFLEXOLOGY · 31

Lower Arch

Bowel and digestive problems, including abdominal cramping, irritable bowel syndrome, Crohn's disease and diarrhoea, can be assisted through stimulation of the reflex points on the lower arch.

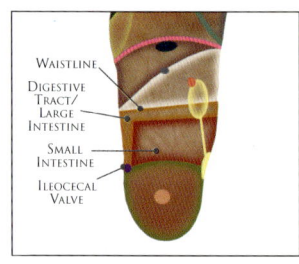

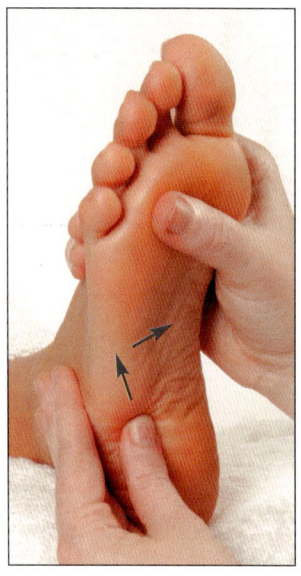

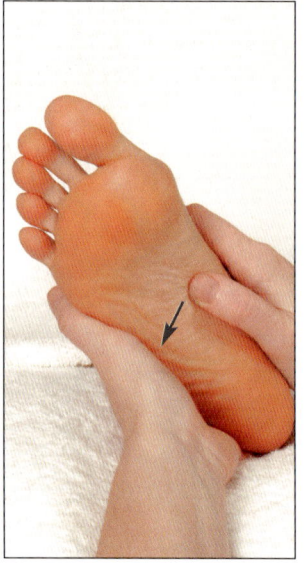

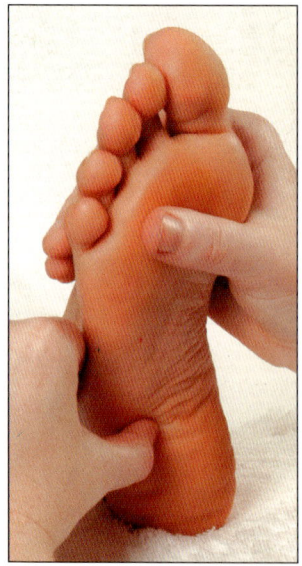

Digestive Tract/Large Intestine Reflex R

Caterpillar along the digestive tract, up to the waistline and across, always moving in the same direction. Repeat 3 times.

Small Intestine Reflex B

When doing reflexology on the left foot, perform the digestive tract/large intestine reflex before commencing the small intestine reflex.

Caterpillar horizontally across the small intestine reflex, starting at the inside (or medial side) of the foot. Repeat 3 times, or until the reflex has been completely covered.

Ileocecal Valve Reflex R

Using your thumb, perform the hook in and up method on the ileocecal valve reflex. Repeat this motion 3 times.

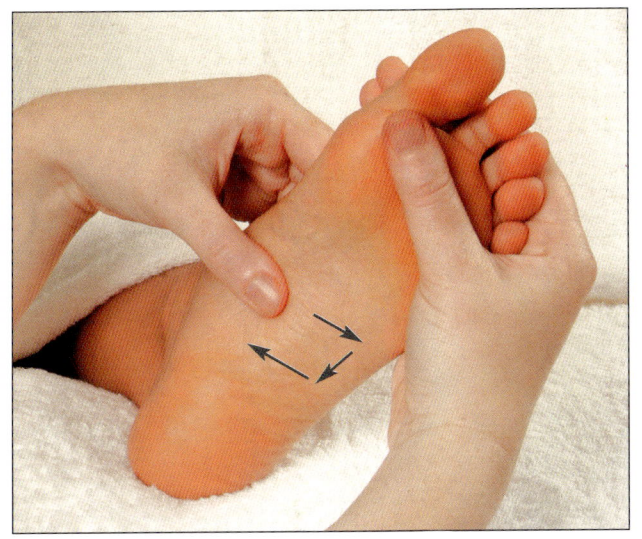
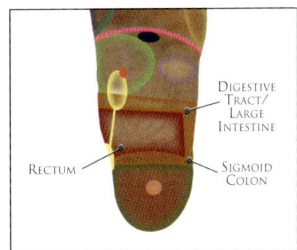

Digestive Tract/Large Intestine Reflex

Support the ankle with your holding hand while working with the other hand. Caterpillar across the digestive tract reflex along the waistline, down along the transverse colon and across the descending colon. Always move in the same direction along the reflex. You can change hands for easier access to the reflex. Repeat 3 times.

Next, perform the small intestine reflex on page 32 before moving on to the sigmoid colon reflex.

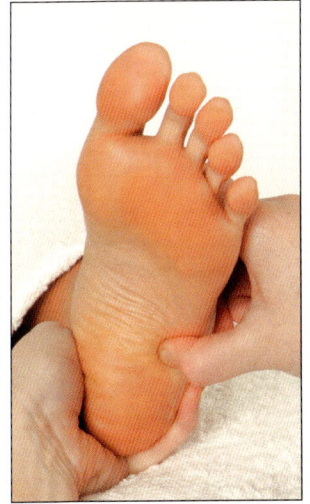

Sigmoid Colon Reflex

Using your thumb, perform the hook in and up method on the sigmoid colon reflex. Repeat this motion 3 times.

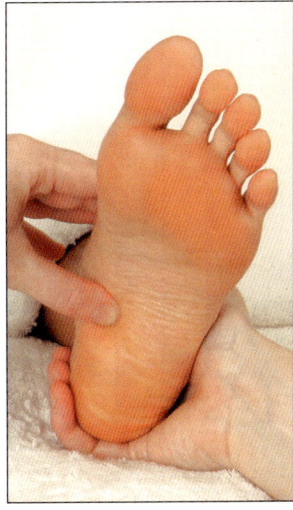

Rectum Reflex

Using your thumb, perform the hook in and up method on the rectum reflex. Repeat this motion 3 times.

Heel

The heel area relates to the pelvic region and sciatic nerve. Reflexology on this area will help with pelvic problems and sciatic and lower back conditions.

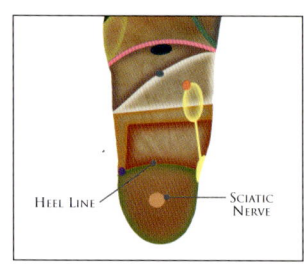

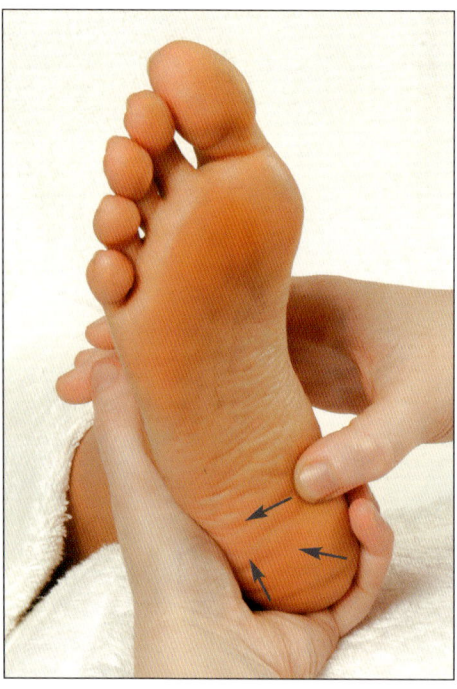

Using the caterpillar technique on the sciatic nerve reflex

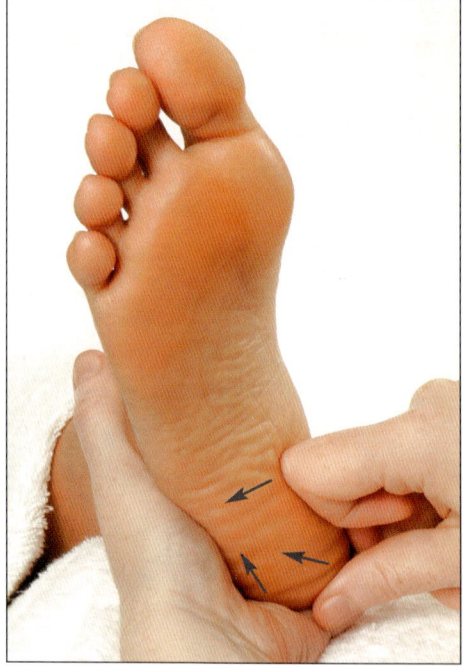

Using the knuckles technique on the sciatic nerve reflex

Sciatic Nerve Reflex B

Support the ankle with your holding hand while working with the other hand. To work this area, caterpillar over the whole heel, covering it first horizontally, then vertically and finally diagonally. Repeat 3 times.

If your partner has thick skin in this area, you can use your knuckles, remembering to work to your partner's tolerance.

INSIDE OF THE FEET

The reflexes on the inside of the feet can be stimulated for menopausal, menstrual, fertility and prostate problems.

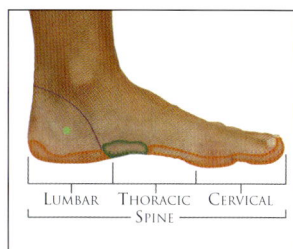

LUMBAR | THORACIC | CERVICAL
— SPINE —

Spinal Twist Relaxer

Hold the lower arch of the foot in both hands (fingers on the dorsal aspect, thumbs on the plantar, or sole) and gently twist back and forward in opposite directions, as if wringing out a cloth. Perform two of these in the same spot and then move both hands up the foot towards the toes. Repeat the sequence until you've covered the length of the spinal reflex.

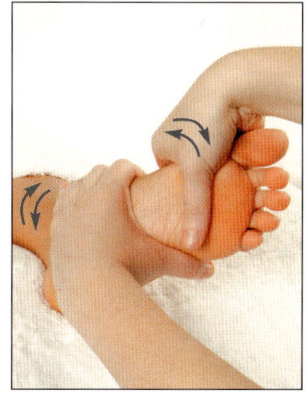
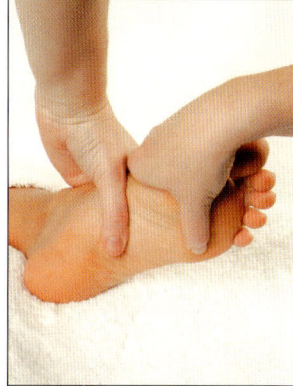

Vertebral Push Relaxer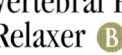

Hold your thumb against the big toe at the top of the spinal reflex and push the foot gently against the thumb. Release the hold and move your thumb down the spinal reflex slightly. Repeat the pushing movement. Continue this sequence down the whole spinal reflex to the heel, using the pushing movement. Picture in your mind that you are working each vertebra of the spine in turn.

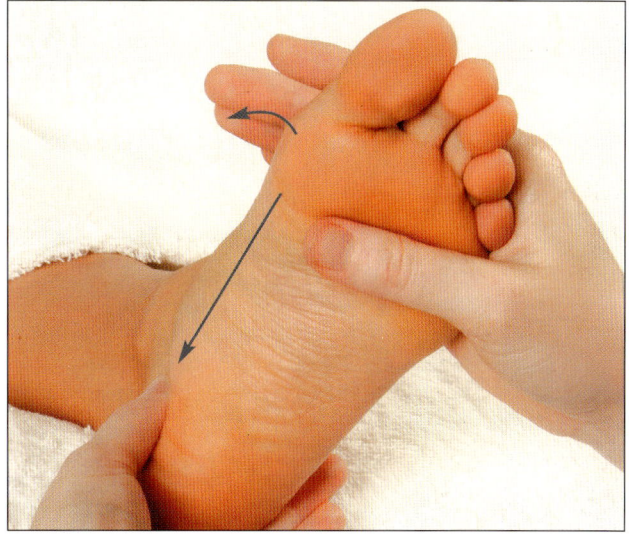

SIMPLY REFLEXOLOGY · 35

Inside of the Feet *(continued)*

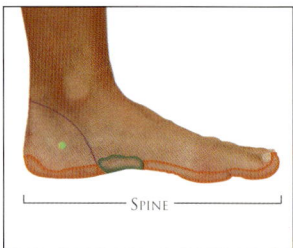

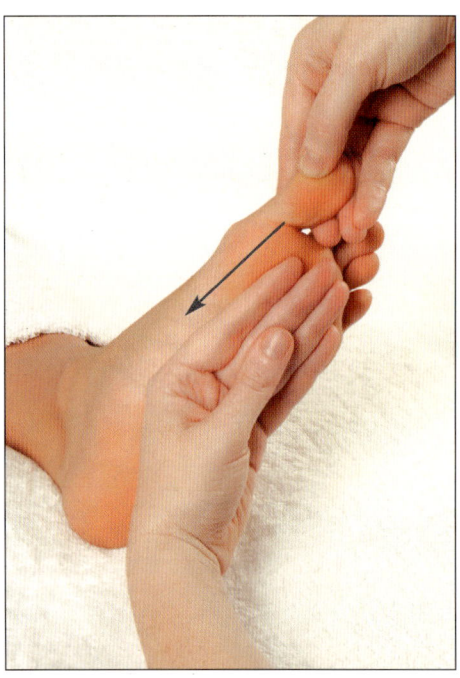

Holding the foot to caterpillar down the spinal reflex

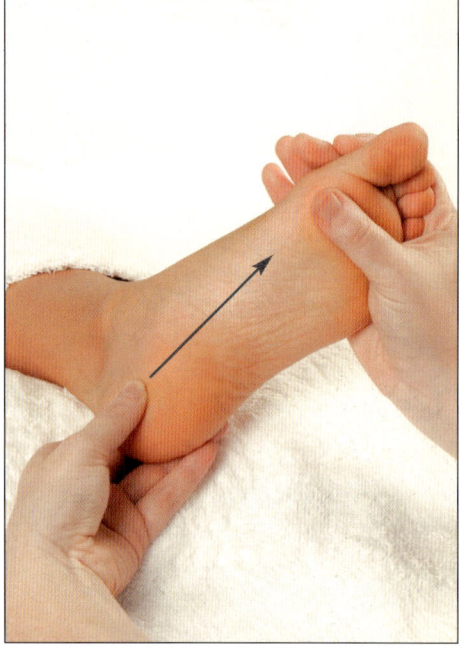

Holding the foot to caterpillar up the spinal reflex

Spinal Reflex B

Lay the back of your holding hand against the sole of the foot, your fingers pointing towards the toes. With your other hand, caterpillar from the big toe in small movements slowly down the spinal reflex, which follows the bony edge of the foot.

Change your hands over, with your holding hand supporting the toes. With your other hand, caterpillar slowly back up the spinal reflex along the bony edge of the foot in small movements, from the heel to the big toe. Repeat this sequence 3 times.

UTERUS/
PROSTATE
GLAND

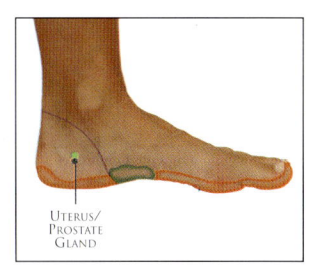

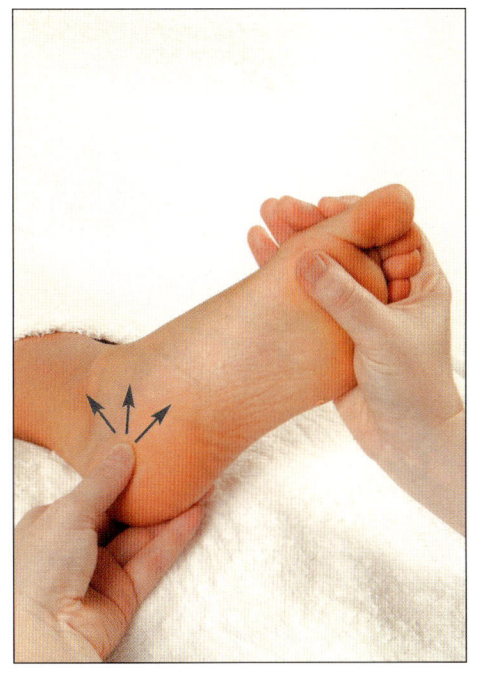

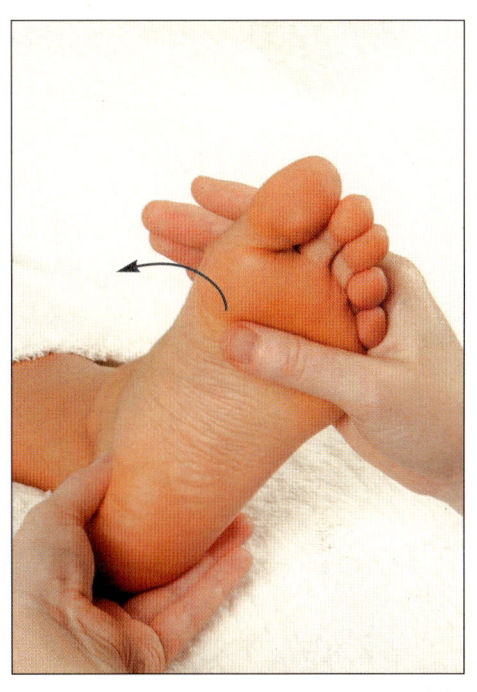

Uterus/Prostate Gland Reflex B

Hold the foot supporting the toes with your holding hand and working with your other hand. If you can, and if it's not uncomfortable for your partner, tilt the foot away from you so that you have easier access to the medial side of the foot.

Using the caterpillar technique, cover the whole inside of the heel area, first horizontally, then vertically and finally diagonally with your thumb. Repeat 3 times each way.

Locate the uterus/prostate gland reflex halfway along an imaginary line running from the edge of the heel to the ankle bone. Place your thumb on the reflex and, with your other hand, hold the foot supporting the toes. Lift the foot over on to your thumb in a rotating motion. Repeat this sequence 3 times.

Outside of the Feet

The ovaries/testes reflex on the outside of the feet relates to infertility, menstrual irregularities, ovarian cysts and menopause. The hip/knee reflex is stimulated to help heal sports injuries and all joint, cartilage and ligament problems.

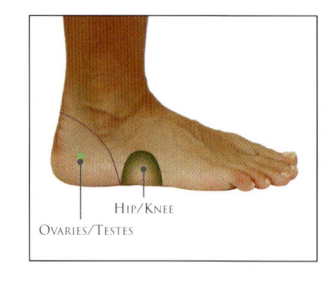

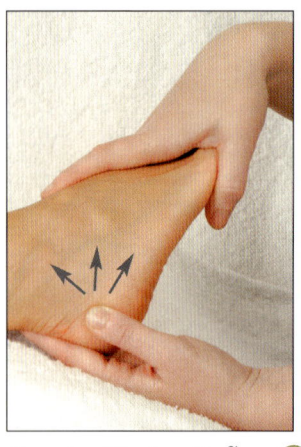

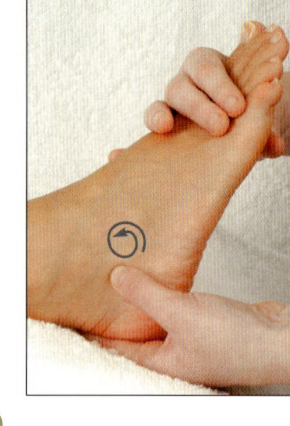

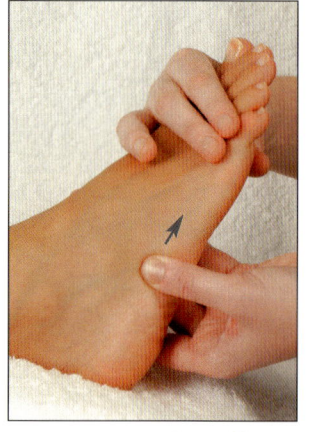

Ovaries/Testes Reflex B

Hold the foot supporting the toes with your holding hand and working with your other hand. If you can, and if it's not uncomfortable for your partner, tilt the foot medially so you have easier access to the lateral side or outside of the foot.

Using the caterpillar technique, cover the whole outside of the heel area, first horizontally, then vertically and finally diagonally, with your thumb. Repeat 3 times each way. If necessary, you can swap hands for easier access to the area.

Locate the ovaries/testes reflex halfway along an imaginary line running from the edge of the heel to the ankle bone. Place your thumb on the reflex and gently rotate it. Repeat this 3 times.

Hip/Knee Reflex B

Caterpillar your thumb across the hip/knee reflex, making sure to completely cover the area. Repeat 3 times.

Top of the Feet

The top of the feet encompass reflex points that aid lung conditions, breast tenderness due to pre-menstrual tension, infertility and reproductive problems. These reflex points will also help fight infection, detox your body and reduce swelling of the feet.

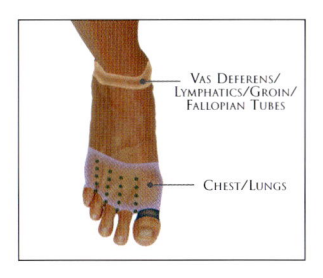

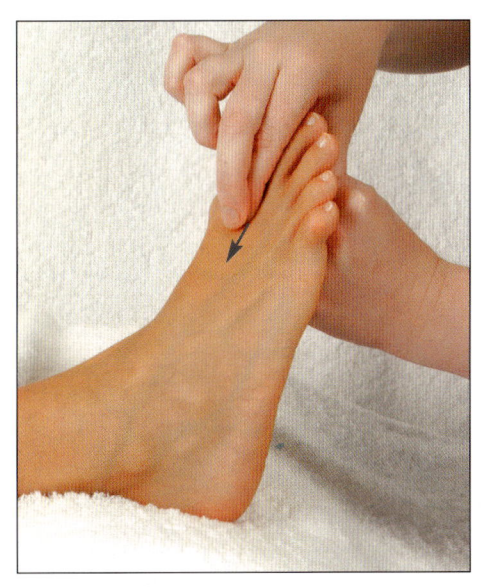

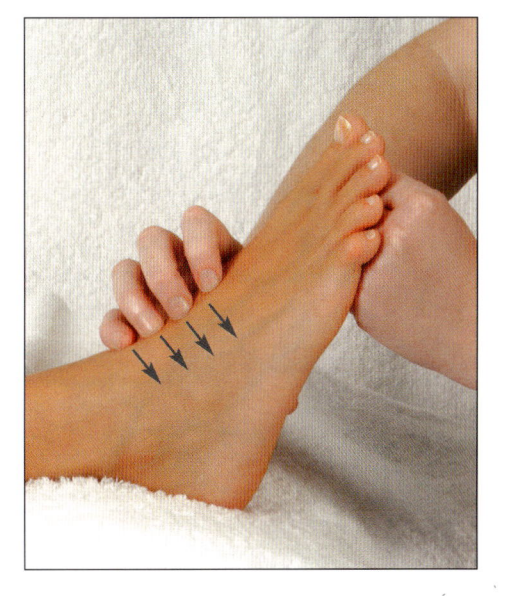

Vas Deferens/Lymphatics/Groin/Fallopian Tubes

Chest/Lungs

Chest Reflex B

Apply more cream to the top of the foot, as the thin skin in this area is more delicate than on the sole of the foot.

Press your fist into the ball of the foot to enable the metatarsal channels to spread slightly. Place your middle finger on top of the index finger and gently caterpillar down each metatarsal channel starting from the big toe, moving out to the little toe. Change hands and repeat the sequence, starting from the little toe and moving in to the big toe. Repeat the whole series 3 times each way.

Vas Deferens/Lymphatics/Groin/Fallopian Tubes Reflex B

Continue supporting the foot from behind with your holding hand fist. Starting from the inside of the foot, caterpillar with the four fingers of the other hand held together. Move horizontally across the foot to the outside. This technique is known as 'marching armies'. Repeat 3 times.

Important note: Avoid performing reflexology on the reproductive area during pregnancy.

Inner Arch

Use reflexology on the inner arch for bladder and kidney infections, fluid retention, bed-wetting and incontinence, glaucoma, skin conditions, blood pressure and arthritis.

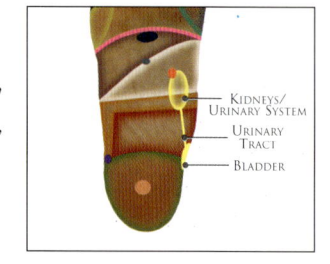

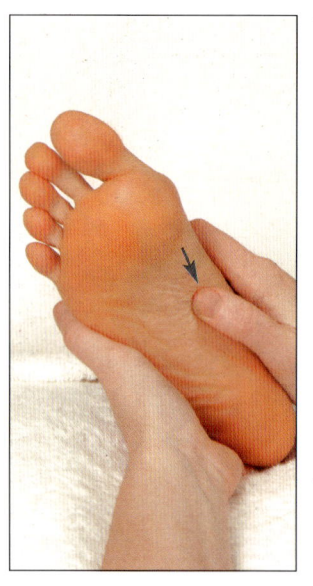

KIDNEYS/URINARY SYSTEM
URINARY TRACT
BLADDER

Kidneys/Urinary System Reflex B

Hold the right foot in your left hand, supporting the toes with your left hand and working with your right hand. When performing reflexology on the left foot, reverse your hands. If you can, and if it's not uncomfortable for your partner, tilt the foot laterally.

Caterpillar down the kidneys/urinary system reflex using your thumb. Repeat 3 times.

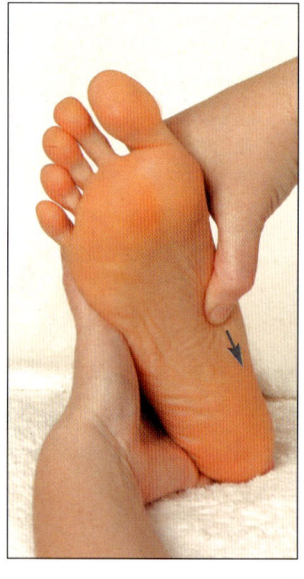

Urinary Tract Reflex B

Maintaining the same holding position, caterpillar with your thumb down the urinary tract reflex, which runs from the kidneys to the bladder reflexes. Repeat 3 times.

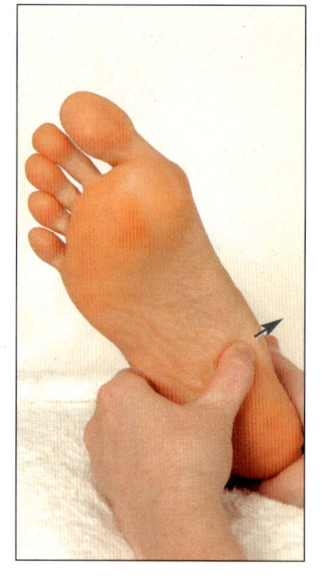

Bladder Reflex B

Caterpillar your thumb horizontally across the bladder reflex area, working from the lateral to the medial side of the foot. Repeat 3 times.

40 · SIMPLY REFLEXOLOGY

Finishing Sequence

Any toxins that have been released during the session will be dispersed with the exercises in the finishing sequence. It is therefore advisable that your partner drinks a glass of water at the end of the session to flush out the toxins.

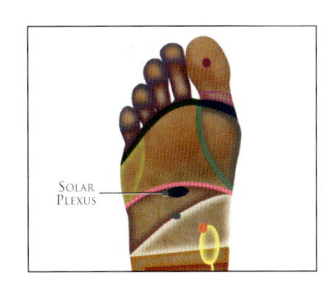

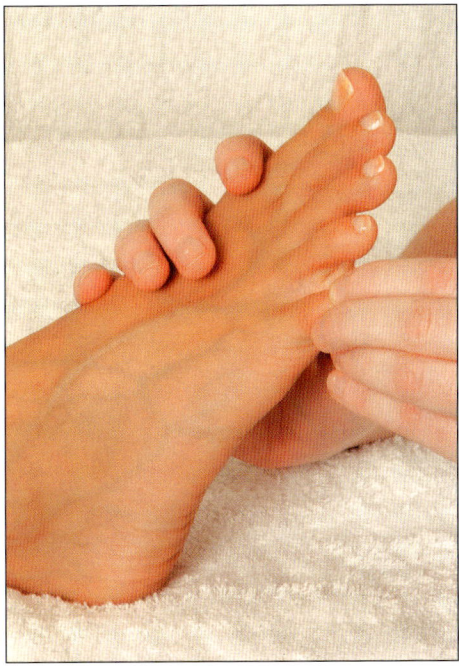

SOLAR PLEXUS

Wiggle Toes B

Perform this sequence on the right foot before commencing reflexology on the left foot. When you finish the left foot, perform this sequence before moving on to the solar plexus hold.

Support the foot with your holding hand. Starting with the little toe, grasp each toe in turn and gently rotate it 3 times in a clockwise direction and then 3 times in an anti-clockwise direction. Gently sweep both hands down the dorsal aspect of the feet. Repeat 3 times.

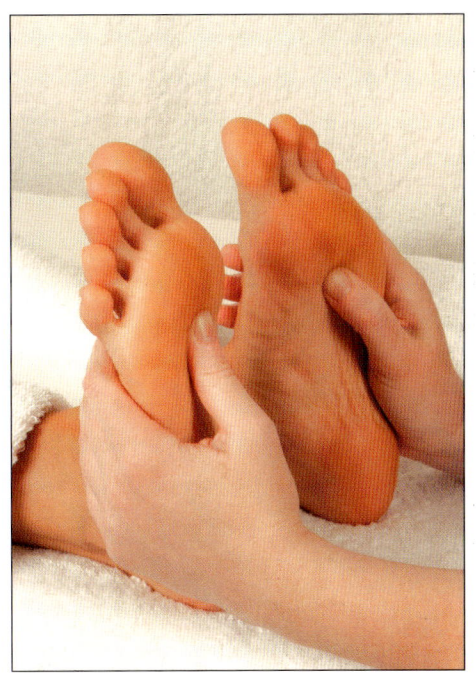

Solar Plexus Hold B

Perform this sequence only after you have completed reflexology on both feet.

Place your thumbs on the solar plexus reflex of each foot. Press in and hold for a count of 3, then release.

Once you have finished, rub your partner's feet with a towel to get rid of any excess cream – this also helps your partner feel more refreshed and revived after a session.

Whole Sequence - Right Foot ®

Perform all relaxers on the right foot before commencing the right foot reflexology sequence.

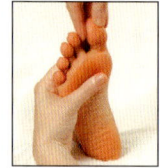

1 Head Reflex
2 Thyroid Gland Reflex 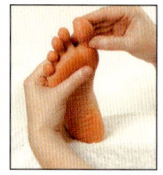
3 Neck Reflex 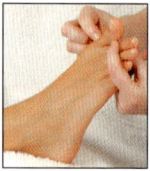
4 Pituitary Gland Reflex 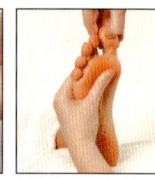
5 Head of the Toe Reflex 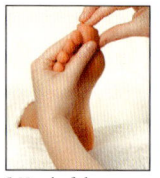
6 Sinus Reflex 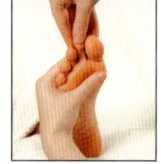
7 Shoulder Reflex 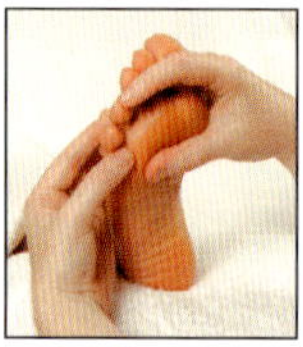
8 Heart Reflex 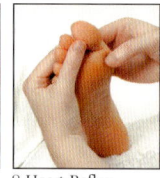
9 Bronchial Tract Reflex 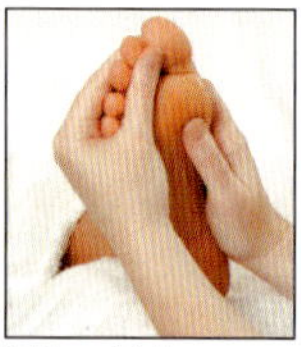
10 Lung Reflex 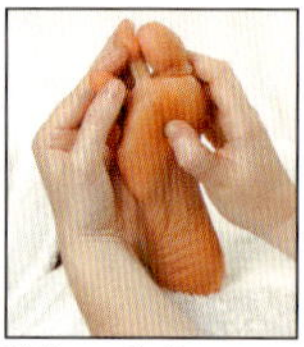
11 Metatarsal Wiggling 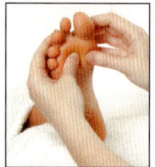
12 Diaphragm Line 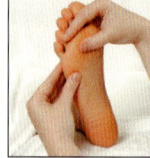
13 Liver Reflex 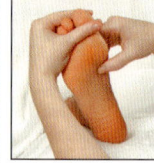
14 Gall Bladder Reflex 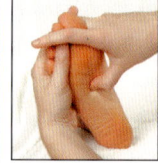
15 Adrenal Gland Reflex 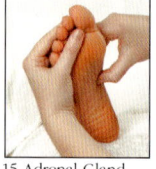
16 Digestive Tract/Large Intestine Reflex 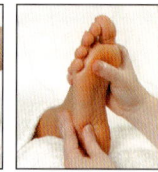
17 Small Intestine Reflex 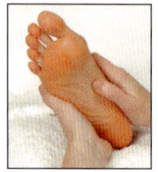
18 Ileocecal Valve Reflex 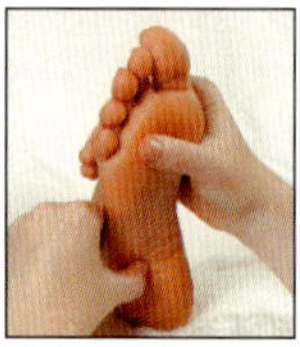
19 Sciatic Nerve Reflex 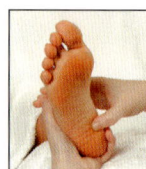
20 Spinal Twist Relaxer 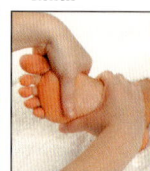
21 Vertebral Push Relaxer 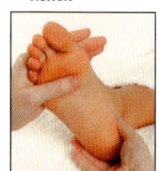
22 Spinal Reflex 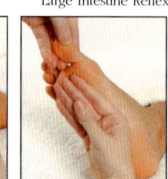
23 Uterus/Prostate Gland Reflex 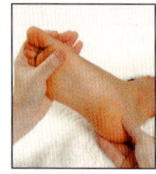
24 Ovaries/Testes Reflex 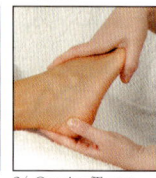
25 Hip/Knee Reflex 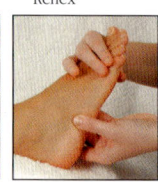
26 Chest Reflex 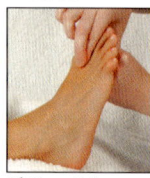
27 Vas Deferens/ Lymphatics/ Groin/Fallopian Tubes Reflex 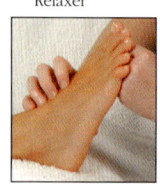
28 Kidneys/Urinary System Reflex 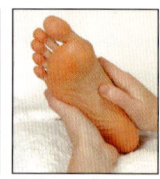
29 Urinary Tract Reflex 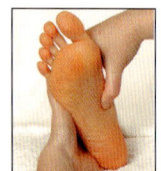
30 Bladder Reflex 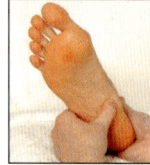
31 Wiggle Toes 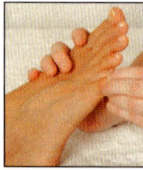

42 · SIMPLY REFLEXOLOGY

Whole Sequence - Left Foot ⓛ

Perform all relaxers on the left foot before commencing the left foot reflexology sequence.

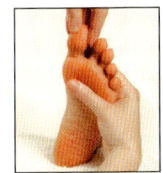

1 Head Reflex

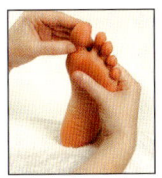

2 Thyroid Gland Reflex

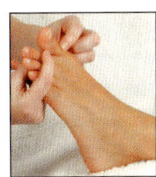

3 Neck Reflex

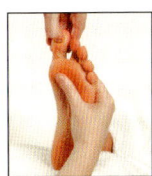

4 Pituitary Gland Reflex

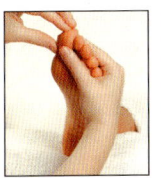

5 Head of the Toe Reflex

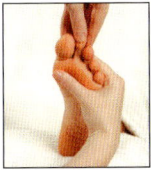

6 Sinus Reflex

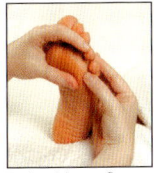

7 Shoulder Reflex

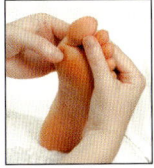

8 Heart Reflex

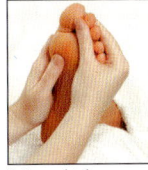

9 Bronchial Tract Reflex

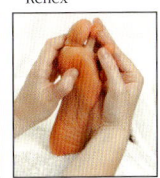

10 Lung Reflex

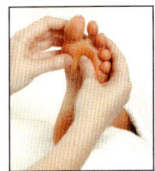

11 Metatarsal Wiggling

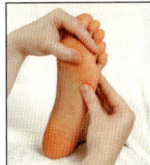

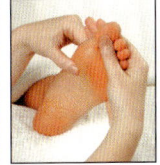

12 Diaphragm Line

13 Stomach and Spleen Reflexes

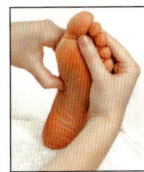

14 Adrenal Gland Reflex

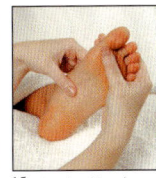

15 Digestive Tract/ Large Intestine Reflex

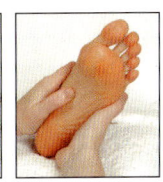

16 Small Intestine Reflex

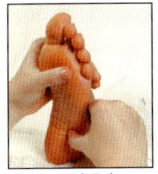

17 Sigmoid Colon Reflex

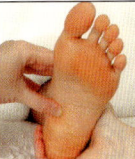

18 Rectum Reflex

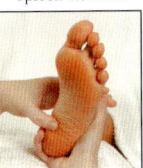

19 Sciatic Nerve Reflex

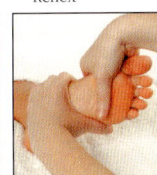

20 Spinal Twist Relaxer

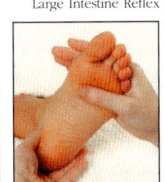

21 Vertebral Push Relaxer

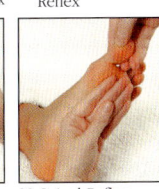

22 Spinal Reflex

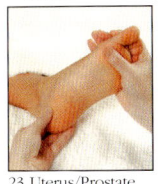

23 Uterus/Prostate Gland Reflex

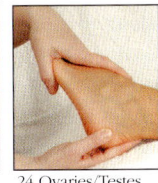

24 Ovaries/Testes Reflex

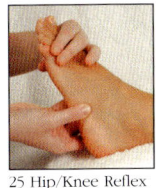

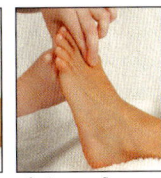

25 Hip/Knee Reflex

26 Chest Reflex

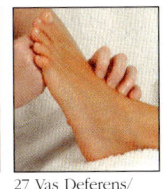

27 Vas Deferens/ Lymphatics/ Groin/Fallopian Tubes Reflex

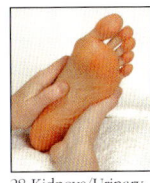

28 Kidneys/Urinary System Reflex

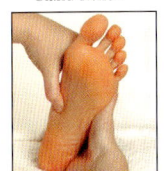

29 Urinary Tract Reflex

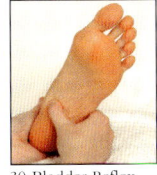

30 Bladder Reflex

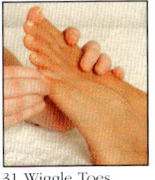

31 Wiggle Toes

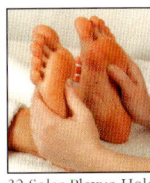

32 Solar Plexus Hold

SIMPLY REFLEXOLOGY · 43

Hands

Anatomy of the Hand

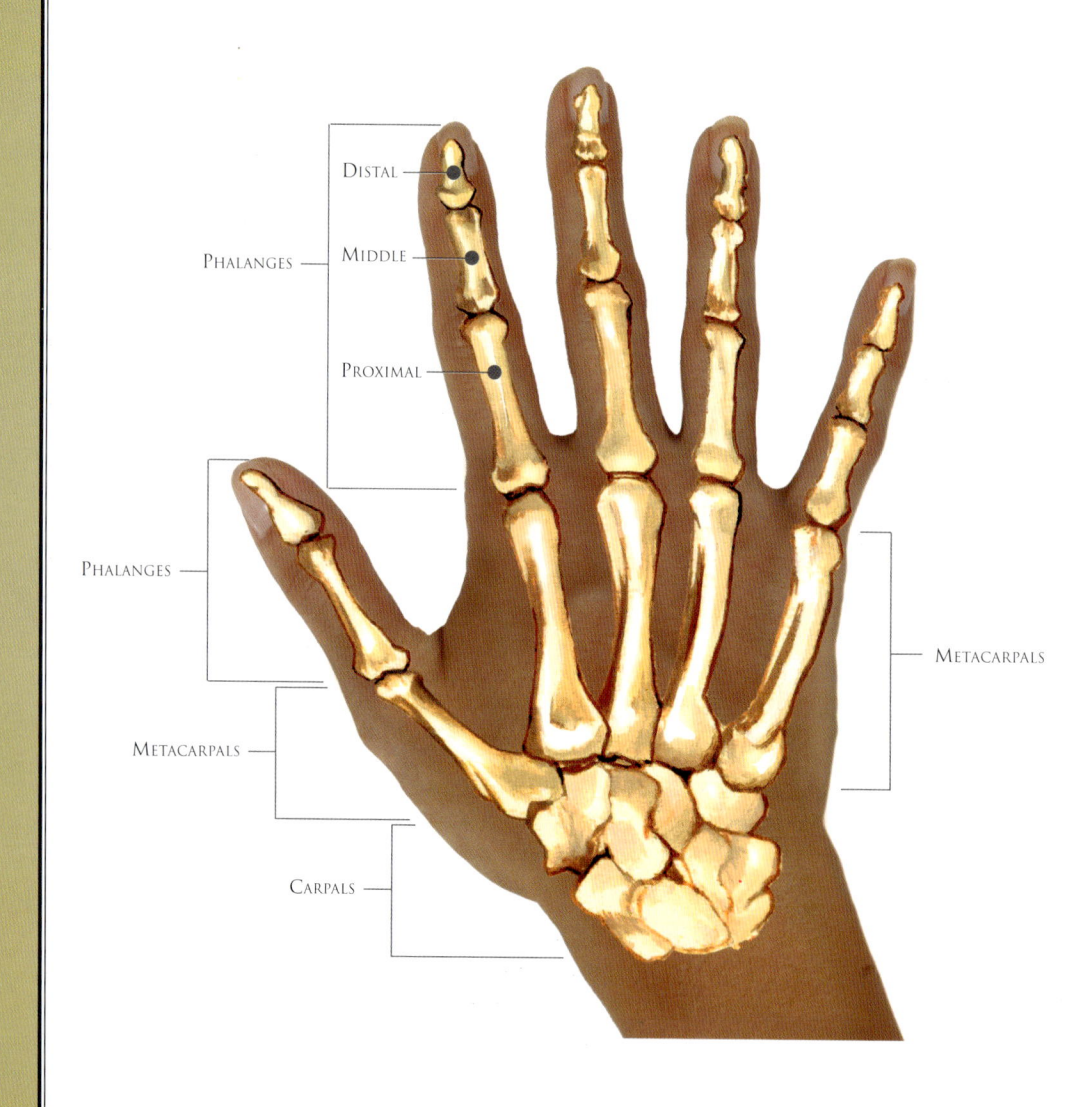

- Phalanges
  - Distal
  - Middle
  - Proximal
- Phalanges
- Metacarpals
- Metacarpals
- Carpals

44 · Simply Reflexology

Reflex Points of the Hands

Palms (Palmar Aspect)

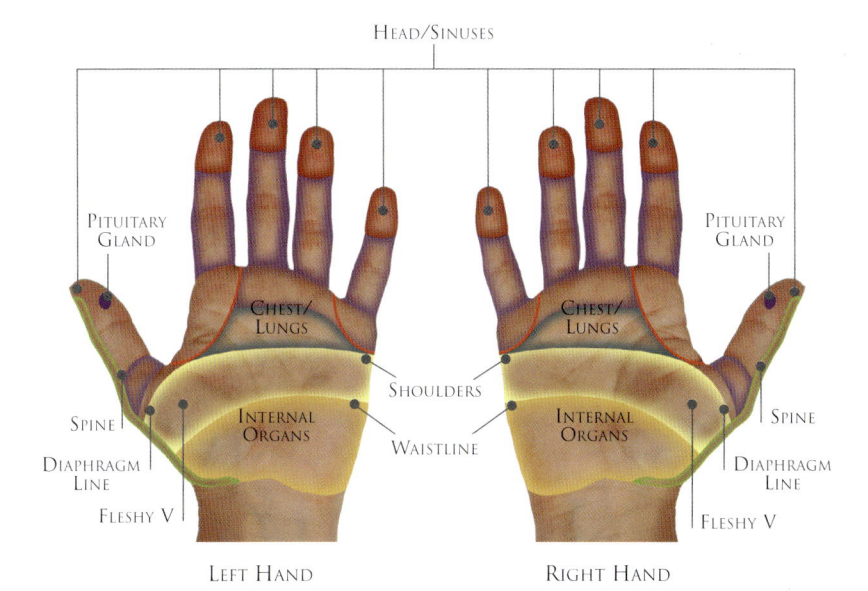

Head/Sinuses

Pituitary Gland

Chest/Lungs

Shoulders

Spine

Internal Organs

Waistline

Diaphragm Line

Fleshy V

Left Hand

Pituitary Gland

Chest/Lungs

Spine

Internal Organs

Diaphragm Line

Fleshy V

Right Hand

Back of the Hands (Dorsal Aspect)

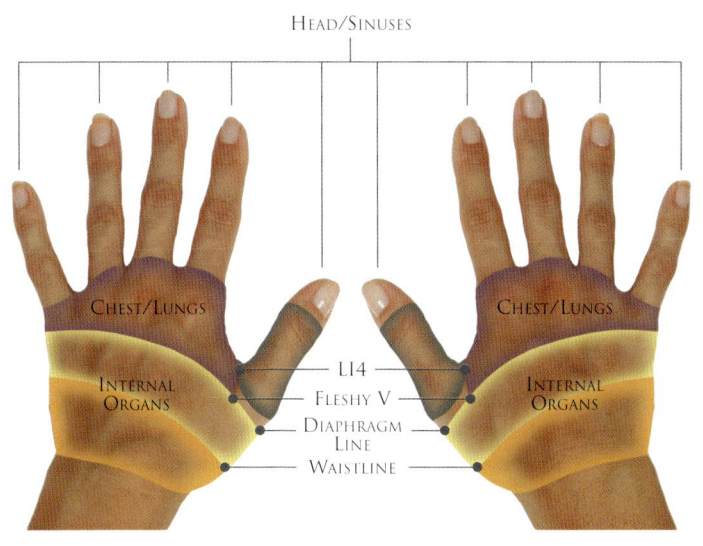

Head/Sinuses

Chest/Lungs

Internal Organs

LI4

Fleshy V

Diaphragm Line

Waistline

Chest/Lungs

Internal Organs

Left Hand

Right Hand

Simply Reflexology · 45

Starting the Session

Loosen your partner's hands in preparation for the session. When treating the hands, it is important to begin with the right hand. Complete the sequences on the right hand, then move onto the left hand in the same manner. Before commencing the session, apply cream to your partner's hands.

Relaxers

Wrist Loosening

Hold your partner's wrist in the palms of both your hands and gently move your palms backwards and forwards. Rock their wrist in your hands for around 10 seconds.

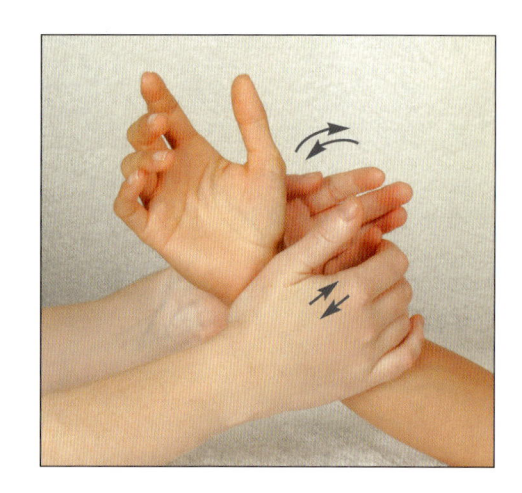

Wrist Circling

Support your partner's hand by placing your fingers under the palm. Use your thumbs to make small circular movements on the wrist, first covering the dorsal area and then turning the hand over to repeat on the palmar (or palm-side) aspect of the wrist. Perform 10 circular movements on each side of the wrist.

Note: If you find you need to support the hand more, you can perform the sequence with one hand, holding your partner's hand with your other hand. Make sure that you double the number of movements to ensure the wrist is completely covered.

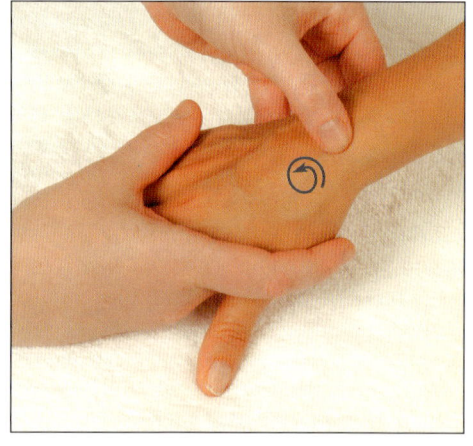

Using one hand to perform wrist circling

Thumb Fanning

Hold your partner's hand with your fingers under the palm. Sweep your thumbs over the dorsal aspect of the hand, using a fanning motion.

Make sure the entire length of your thumbs is in contact with the hand. Perform about 10 sweeping motions, ensuring the whole hand is covered.

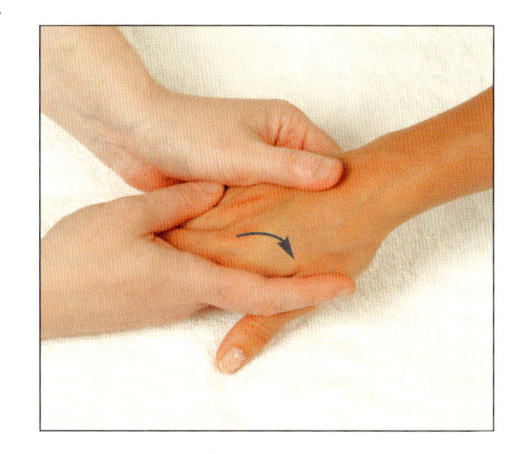

Circular Thumb Rotations

Hold your partner's hand with your holding hand, their palm facing up. With your other hand, make small circular motions over the palm, using your thumb. Ensure you cover the whole palm.

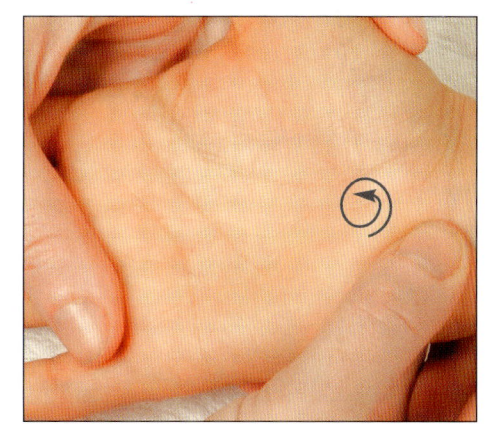

Metacarpal Spreading

With both your hands, hold your partner's hand with the palm facing downwards. Using your thumbs, gently apply pressure to the middle of the back of the hand. As you apply pressure, gently pull the outer edges of the hand upwards and out, spreading the palm of the hand and the metacarpals. Hold for a few seconds, then release. Repeat 3 times.

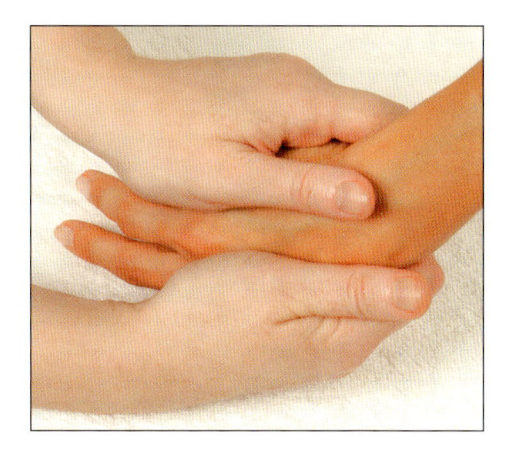

Diaphragm Relaxer

As with the diaphragm relaxer performed on the feet, the hand diaphragm relaxer is excellent for relieving tension in the body and also aids breathing.

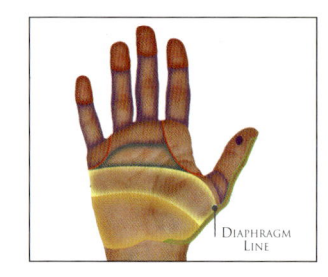

DIAPHRAGM LINE

Step 1

Cup the back of your partner's hand with your holding hand, fingers on the dorsal side and thumb on the palm side. Place the thumb of your other hand on the diaphragm line under the index finger.

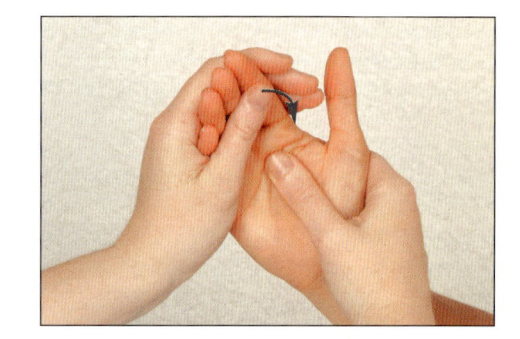

Step 2

Gently pull the hand over your thumb, lifting the hand slightly up and over the thumb. Then lift the hand back off the thumb.

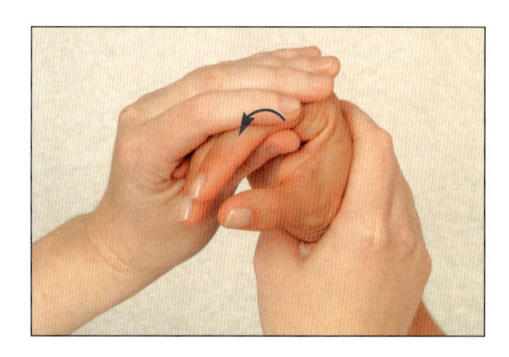

Step 3

Move your thumb slightly along the diaphragm line and repeat step 2. Repeat this sequence in small, gentle movements, covering the whole diaphragm line.

Change your hands over and repeat the sequence going the other way along the diaphragm line.

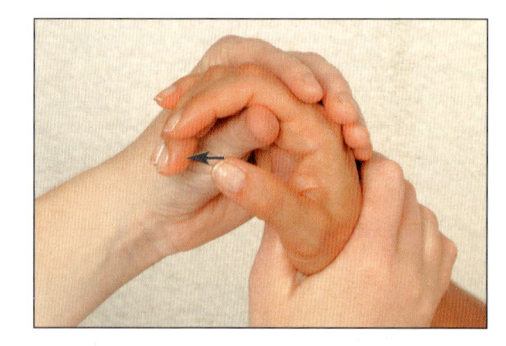

Palms and Front of the Fingers

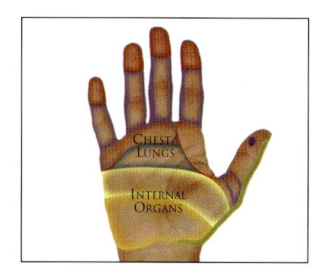

The palms relate to the chest, lungs and internal organs as well as the arms and shoulders. Reflexology on the fingers and thumbs helps with head, eye, ear, sinus, spine and joint problems.

Palmar

Hold your partner's hand open, with the palm facing up. Place the fingers of your holding hand under their palm. Rest your thumb across the top of their four fingers and your index finger over the bottom of their thumb (so that your thumb and index finger form an 'L' shape).

With the thumb of your main hand, first caterpillar horizontally, then vertically and finally diagonally over your partner's palm, making sure you completely cover the whole palm. Repeat the whole sequence 3 times.

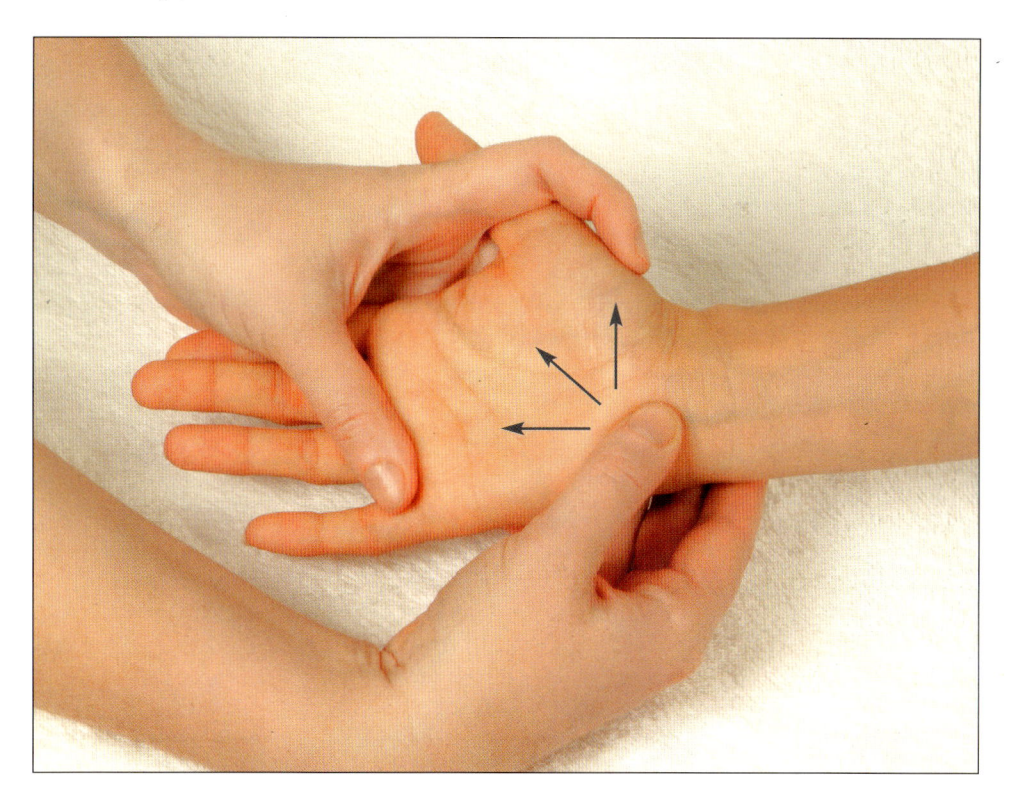

Palms and Front of the Fingers (continued)

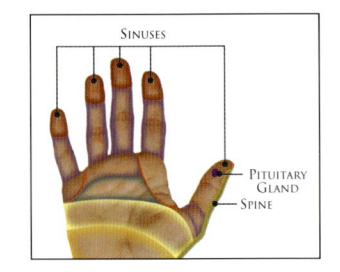

Sinus Reflex

With your supporting hand, hold your partner's hand, with the open palm facing up. Starting at the little finger, caterpillar down each finger and the thumb three times, ensuring that you cover the whole of the palmar aspect of the fingers. If your partner has large fingers, you may need to caterpillar down each finger four times to ensure you cover the whole palmar aspect.

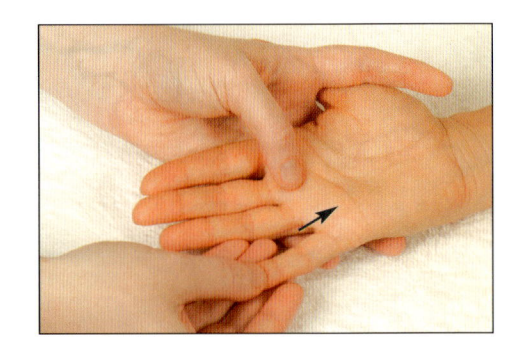

Spinal Reflex

Hold your partner's hand open with the palm facing up. Using your thumb, caterpillar along the spinal reflex, down the thumb and across the heel of the hand. Repeat the sequence 3 times. If it is more comfortable, you can reverse your hands and caterpillar up the reflex from the heel of the hand to the thumb.

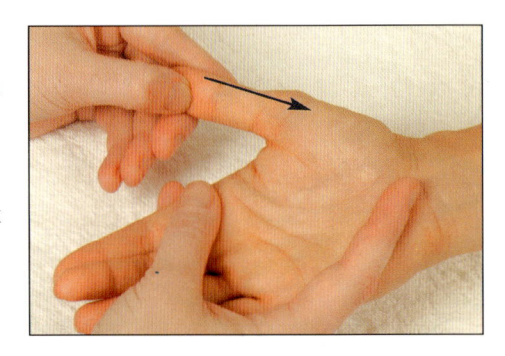

Pituitary Gland Reflex

Maintain the same holding position as the previous sequence. Locate the pituitary gland reflex on the thumbprint swirl of your partner's hand. Using your thumb, perform the hook in and up technique on the reflex. Repeat 3 times.

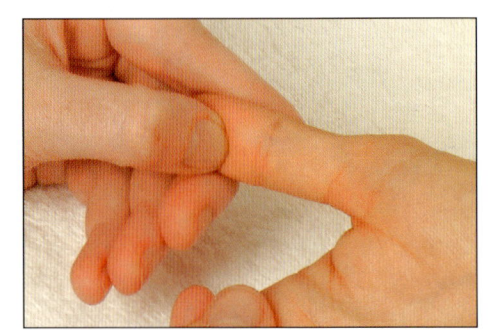

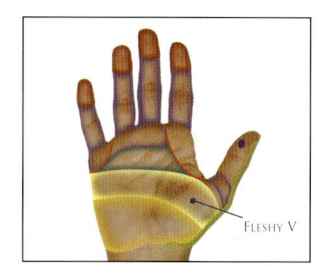

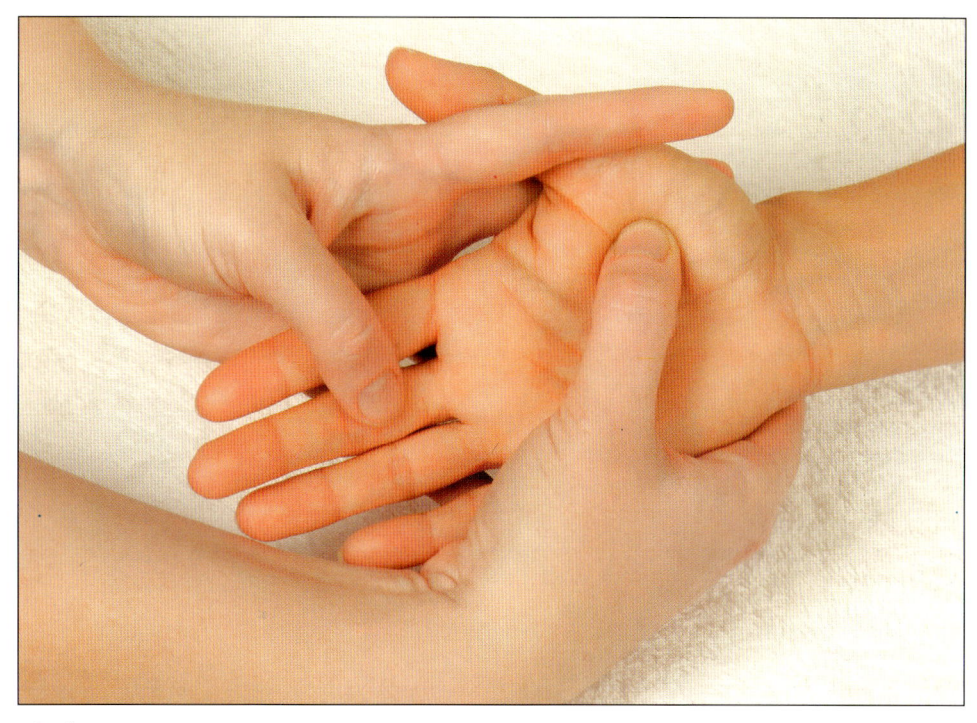

Fleshy V

Locate the fleshy v on the palm of the hand. This is found at the base of the thumb. Cover the fleshy v area, using either small circular motions or the caterpillar movement. Make sure you have covered the whole reflex.

Take care not to press too hard, as this area is quite delicate. This is the largest muscle in the hand, so it's important to work it firmly but not to the discomfort of your partner.

Back of the Hands and Fingers

As well as relating to chest, lungs and internal organs, the back of the hands also relates to the reproductive organs and the hips, legs and knees. The back of the fingers covers the brain, along with the same areas as the front of the fingers.

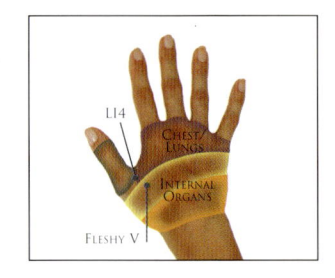

Dorsal

Support your partner's hand with your holding hand, dorsal side facing up. Starting at the little finger, use your thumb to caterpillar from the base of the fingers down each metatarsal channel to the wrist.

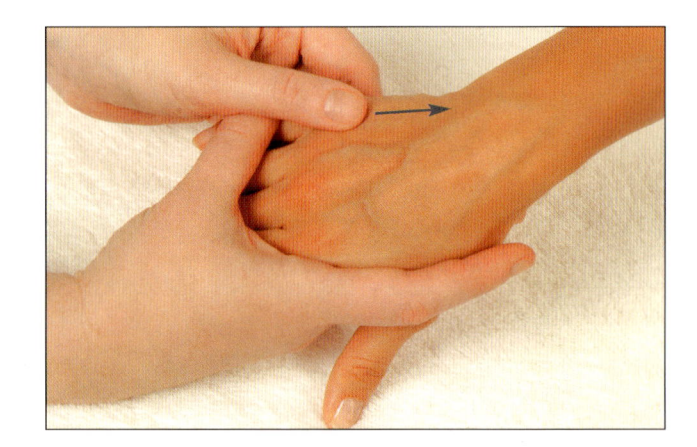

Fleshy V Dorsal

Support your partner's hand with your holding hand, dorsal side facing up. Locate the fleshy v at the base of their thumb. Using your thumb, work over the fleshy v area in small circular movements. Ensure you cover the whole area and be careful not to press too hard, as this area is quite delicate.

This area also incorporates the meridian pressure point large intestine 4 (LI4) which is one of the vital points in traditional Chinese medicine and a great point to use for headaches and stress relief.

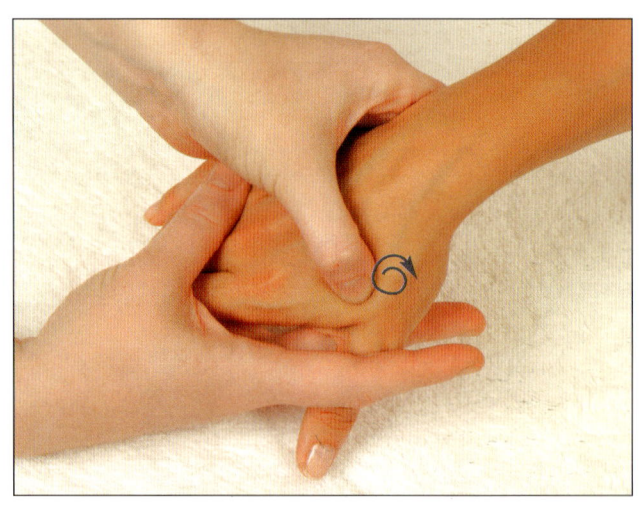

Important note: *Do not stimulate the LI4 area during pregnancy, as it can induce contractions.*

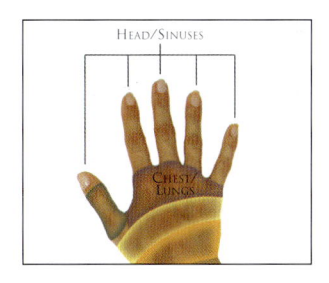

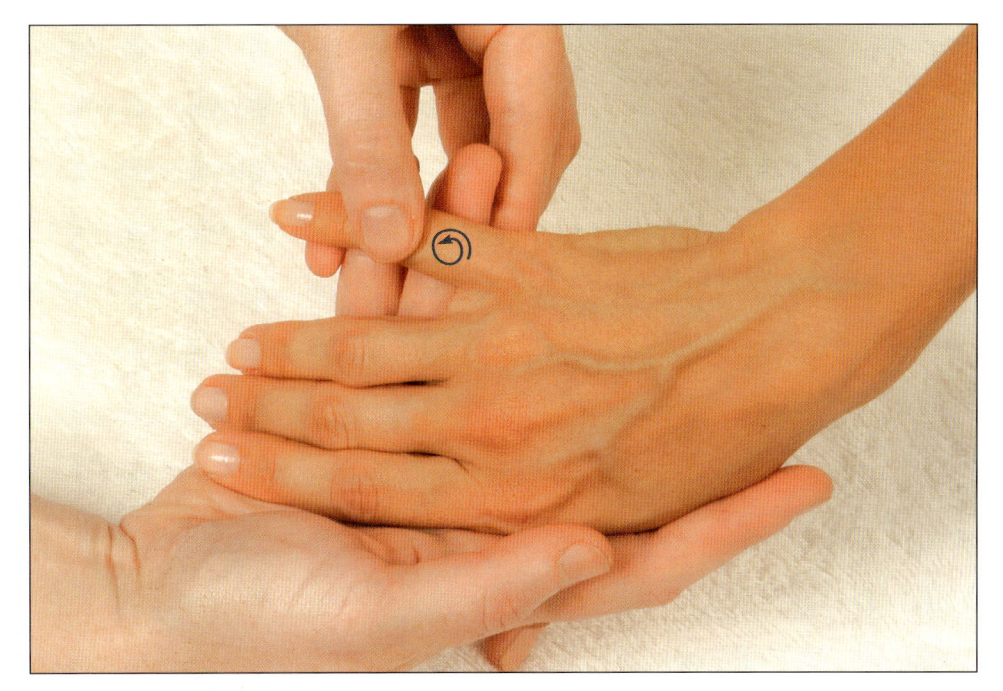

Knuckle Rotations

Hold your partner's hand with the dorsal aspect facing up. Using your thumb, perform three circular rotations on each knuckle. Start at the knuckle at the base of the little finger and work across the hand to the base of the thumb. Then work back across the hand, working both knuckles of each finger until you reach the little finger. You can swap your holding hands based on what feels most comfortable for you.

Gently smooth both your hands down the dorsal aspect of your partner's hand a few times. Exert enough pressure so that your partner's skin drags slightly. You can then finish by performing your choice of relaxer.

Face and Ears

Reflex Points of the Face and Ears

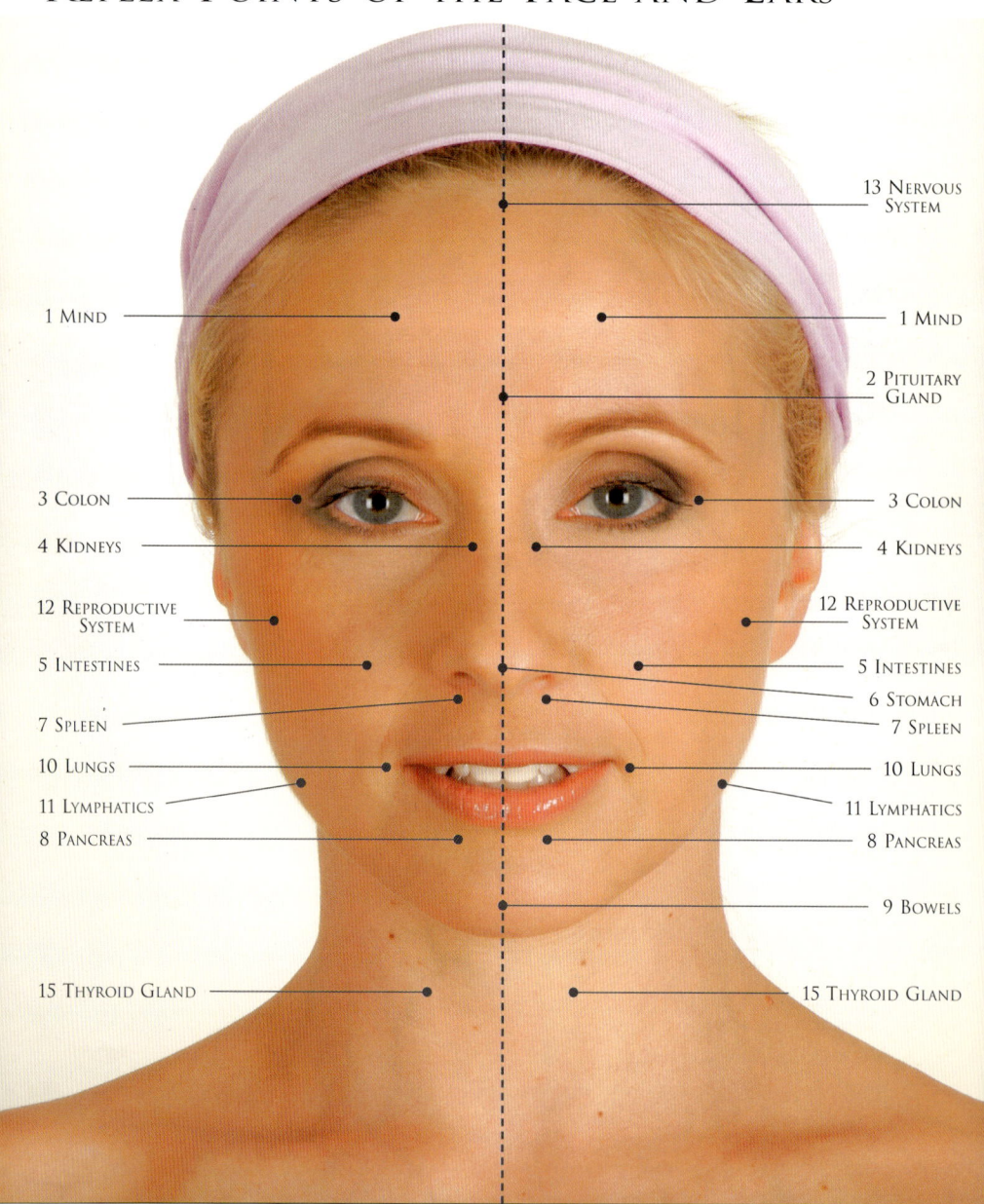

- 1 Mind
- 2 Pituitary Gland
- 3 Colon
- 4 Kidneys
- 5 Intestines
- 6 Stomach
- 7 Spleen
- 8 Pancreas
- 9 Bowels
- 10 Lungs
- 11 Lymphatics
- 12 Reproductive System
- 13 Nervous System
- 15 Thyroid Gland

54 · Simply Reflexology

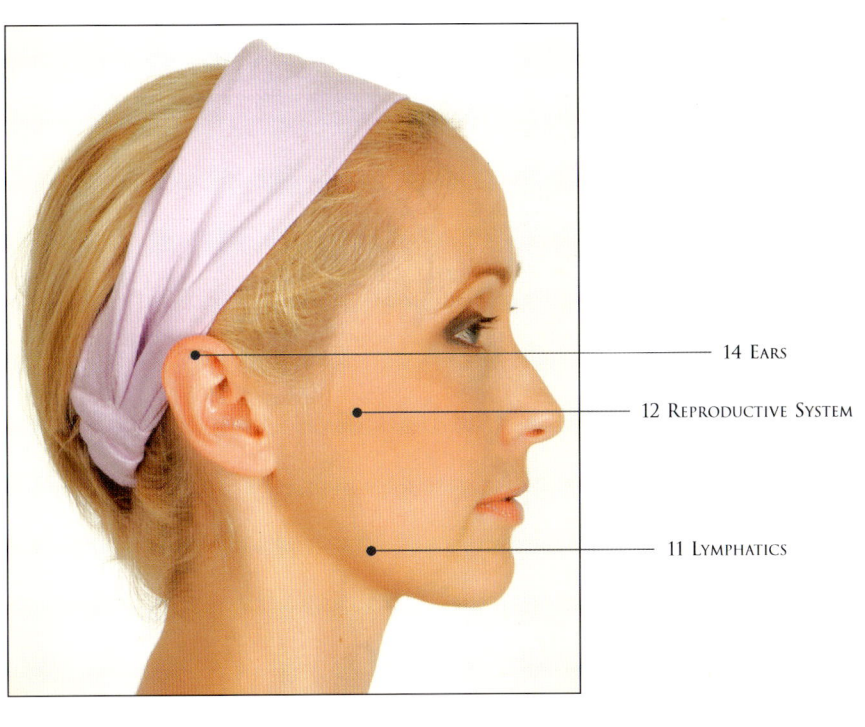

14 Ears
12 Reproductive System
11 Lymphatics

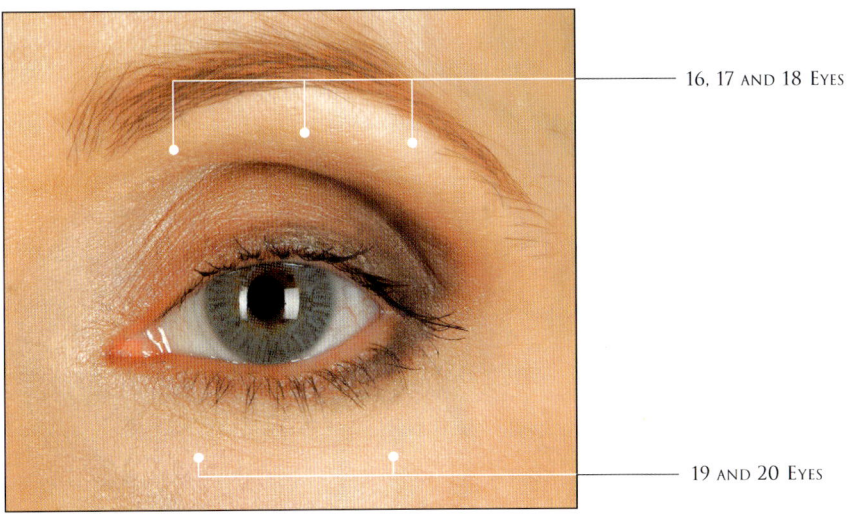

16, 17 and 18 Eyes

19 and 20 Eyes

Simply Reflexology · 55

Starting the Session

Before you start facial and ear reflexology, ask your partner to remove all jewellery, including earrings (you can work around small earrings). Have cotton buds on hand to clean the shell of the ear.

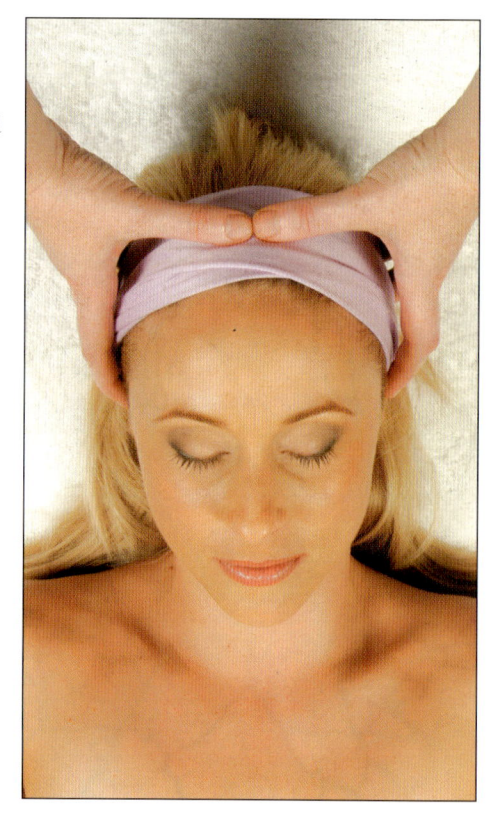

Holding Your Partner's Head

Before you start facial and ear reflexology, it is important that your partner is comfortable with your touch.

Place your hands gently on the head, thumbs side by side on the crown and fingers fanned out to cover the scalp. Hold this position for around 10 seconds.

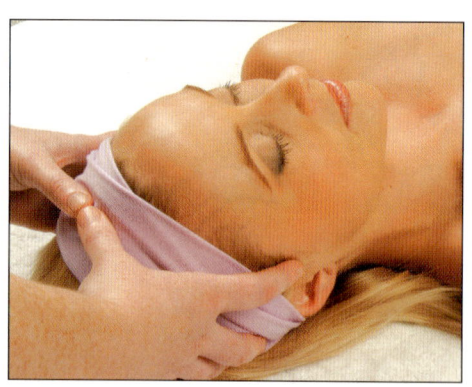

Face

Facial reflexology is used to help alleviate headaches, facial problems, jaw pain, insomnia, dizziness and eye disorders, and for general relaxation and wellbeing.

Facial Reflexology Technique

Facial reflexology is a very gentle therapy, but it is a lot more powerful than it looks. You don't need to apply any pressure when doing reflexology on the face and ears. Just rest the fingers lightly on the face at each reflex point.

Most reflexes on the face are double points; that is, they are mirrored on each side of the face. There are four reflexes that occur as only a single reflex point (pituitary gland, stomach, bowels and nervous system), and they can be found on an imaginary line running down the centre of the face. Spend around a minute performing the movements on each reflex.

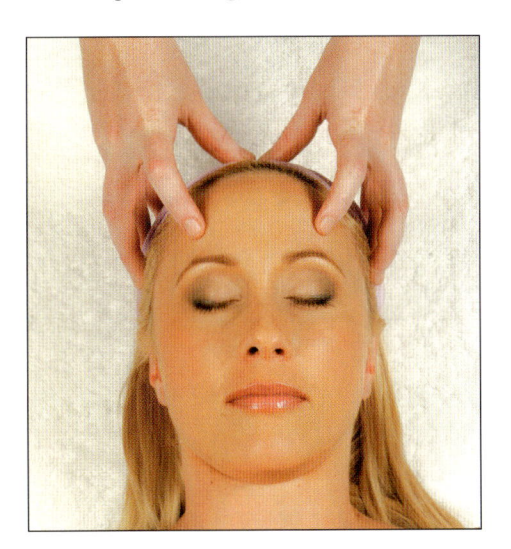

Double Point Techniques

Place your index fingers gently on the reflex points and make small circular motions in an outwards direction, using only the points of the fingertips.

On the pancreas reflex, use the flat of your fingertips instead of the points. Use the flat of two fingertips on the thyroid gland reflex; the index and middle fingers.

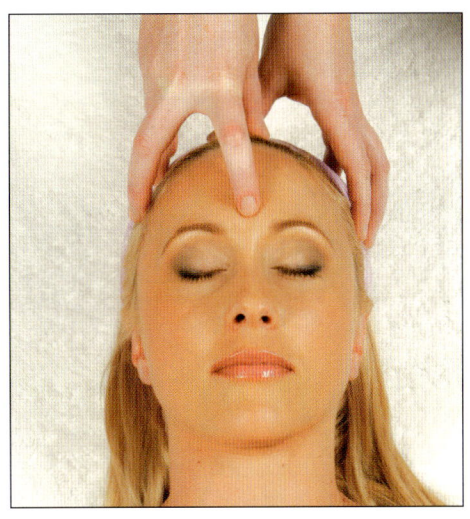

Single Point Technique

Gently place the index fingertip of your main hand on the reflex and make small circular motions with the point. Rest your other hand on top of your partner's head.

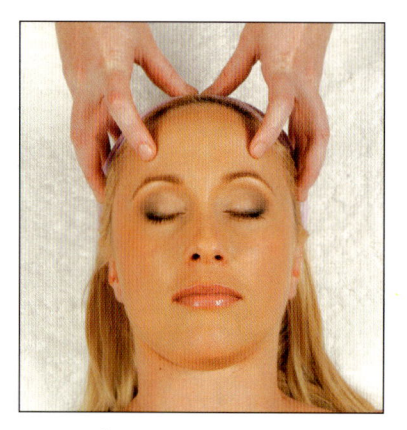

1 Mind

Rest your thumbs on top of your partner's head and place your index fingertip points on the mind reflexes, found on the forehead. Make small circular rotations in an outward direction.

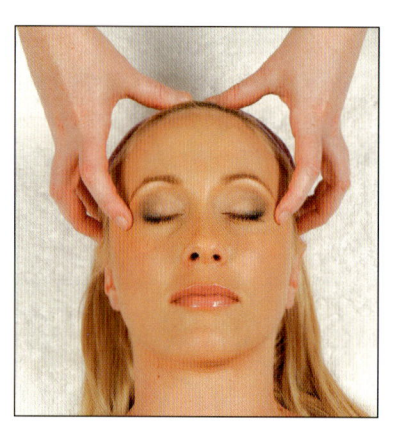

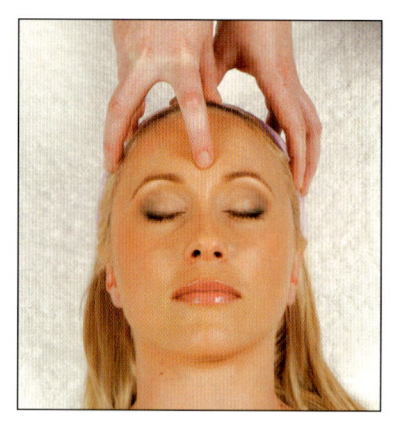

2 Pituitary Gland

With your hands still in the same position on the top of the head, place the index finger of your main hand on the pituitary gland reflex in the centre of the forehead. Repeat the circular motion for around a minute.

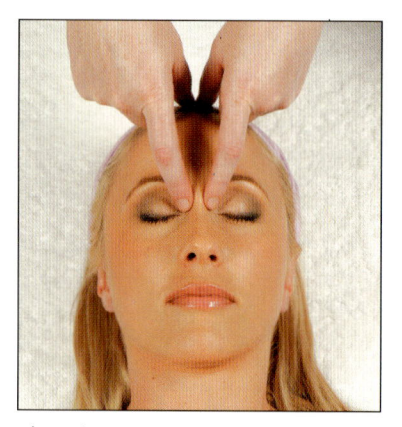

3 Colon

Maintain your hands in the same position on top of the head and locate the colon reflexes next to the eyes. Place your index fingertip points on the reflexes and rotate them gently outwards.

4 Kidneys

Place your thumbs on top of your partner's head. With your fingertip points, locate the kidneys reflexes on the bridge of the nose. Rotate your fingertips outwards for around a minute.

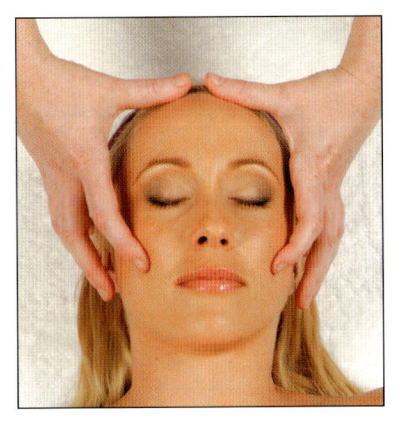

5 Intestines

Rest your thumbs on top of the head and encircle the rest of the head with your hands. Place your fingertip points on the cheeks on the intestines reflexes and rotate them outward.

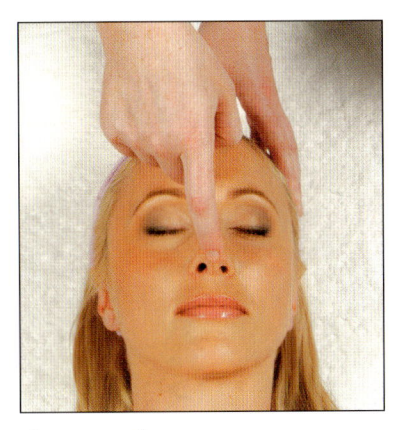

6 Stomach

Place your holding hand on top of the head, thumb in the centre. Locate the stomach reflex with the index fingertip point of your main hand and perform circular rotations on the reflex for around a minute.

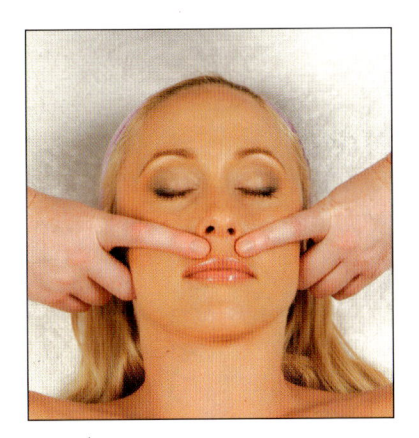

7 Spleen

Locate the spleen reflexes under the nose and rest your index fingertips on the points. Rotate your fingertip points in a circular, outward motion.

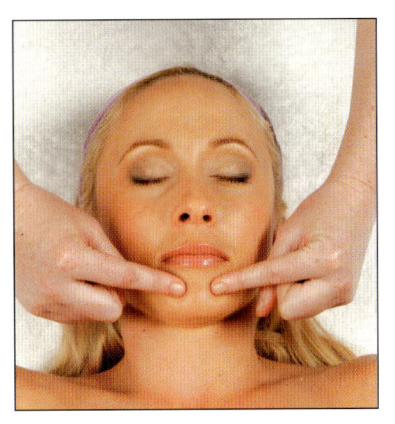

8 Pancreas

Rest the flat of your fingertips on the pancreas reflexes on the chin and gently rotate them in an outward direction.

Simply Reflexology · 59

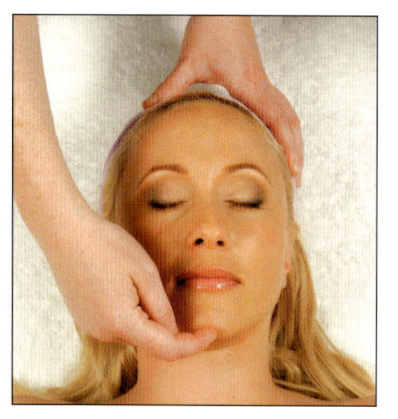

9 Bowels

Rest your holding hand on top of your partner's head. Place the fingertip point of the index finger of your main hand on the bowels reflex, located on the chin. Make small rotations with your fingertip.

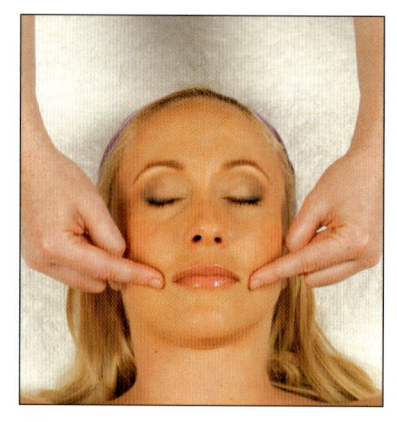

10 Lungs

Locate the lung reflexes next to the mouth. Rest your index fingertip points on the reflexes and rotate them in a circular, outward motion.

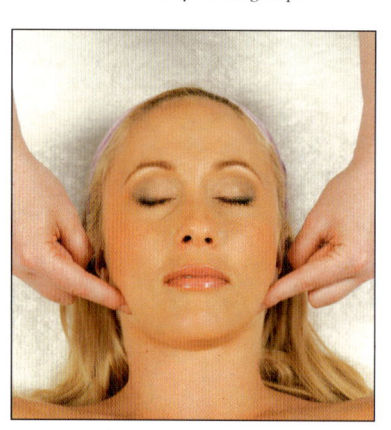

11 Lymphatics

Place your fingertip points on the lymphatic system reflexes on the side of the face. Gently rotate your fingers outward.

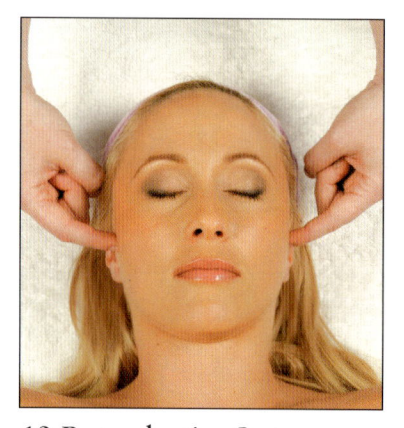

12 Reproductive System

Gently place your fingertip points on the reproductive system reflexes on the cheekbones. Perform gentle rotations in an outward direction.

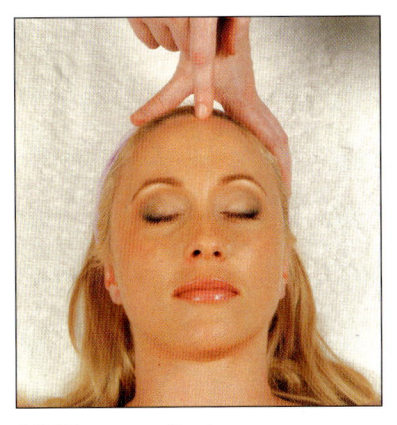

13 Nervous System

Rest your holding hand on top of your partner's head. Place the index fingertip of your main hand on the nervous system reflex, located on top of the forehead. Rotate your fingertip for around a minute.

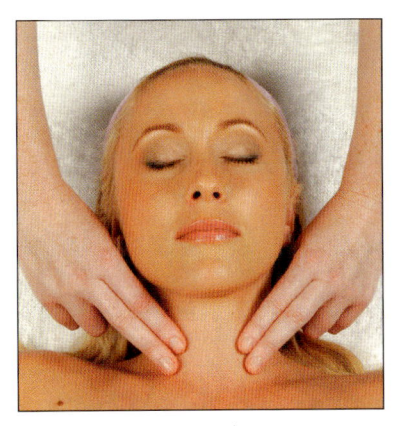

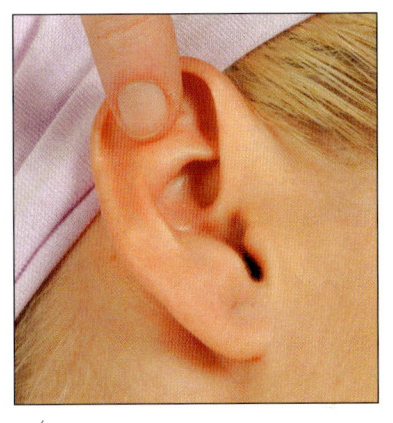

14 Ears

Place your fingertip points on the ear reflexes, located on the upper part of the ear. Perform gentle rotations.

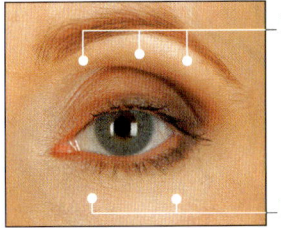

16, 17 AND 18 EYES

19 AND 20 EYES

16, 17, 18, 19 & 20 Eyes

Starting at the point on top of the corner of the eye and working in an outwards direction, gently press on the eye reflex points. Gently press on each reflex for 2 or 3 seconds, and then move on to the next point. As you move around the five main points, lightly touch the skin in between each reflex.

Do not press too hard or use a circular motion, as the skin around the eyes is extremely delicate. Work from the top inside corner of the eye to the outside top corner, and then from the bottom inside corner to the outside bottom corner.

15 Thyroid Gland

Place the flat of your index and middle fingertips on the thyroid gland reflexes, which are found on the neck. Gently rotate your fingers in an outward direction.

SIMPLY REFLEXOLOGY · 61

Ear

Ear reflexology is useful for alleviating a myriad of health problems, including fever, skin disorders, pain, lower back and circulatory problems, toothache, facial paralysis, excessive sweating, hypotension and heart disease.

According to the ancient Chinese, the ear represents the whole body. Imagine the ear as a body curled up in a foetal position, with the head at the ear lobe and the rest of the body curling around to the upper ear.

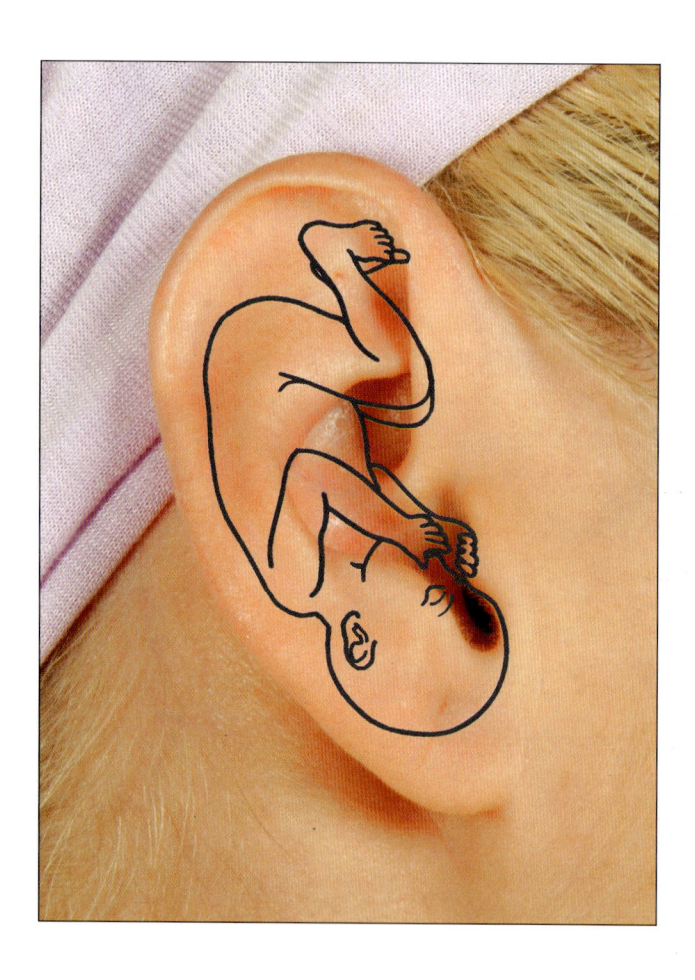

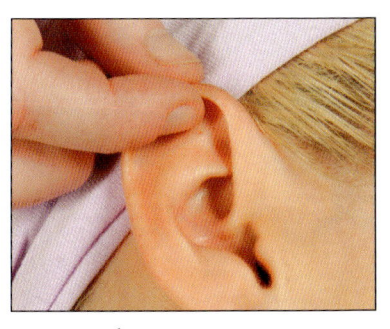

1 Uncurling Ear

Starting at the top of the ear, gently pull on the edge of the ears, as if you are trying to unroll them. Continue this motion, working your way around the edge of the ear until you reach the top of the ear lobe.

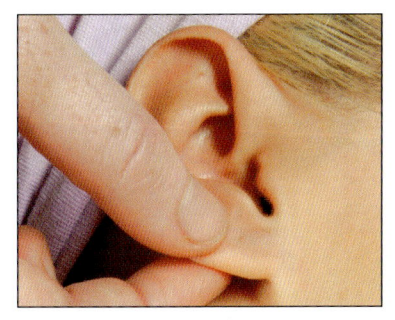

2 Tug Lobes

Gently tug on the ear lobes, rubbing them slightly with your thumb as you pull. Repeat this motion 4 or 5 times.

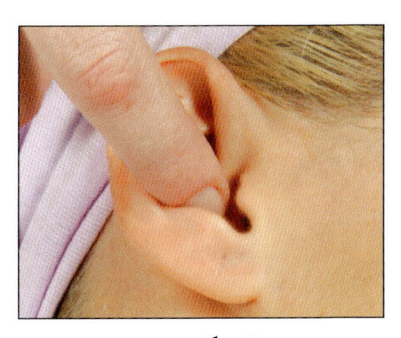

3 Massage Inside Ear

Gently massage the inside of the ear (the hard cartilage protrusion near the ear canal) 3 or 4 times between your thumb and index finger. As the ear is very delicate, you don't need to exert much pressure.

Next, lightly massage the inside of the ear shell with your index finger, using gentle sweeping motions. Work from the ear canal around the top of the ear, down to the lobes and back to the ear canal. Repeat 3 times.

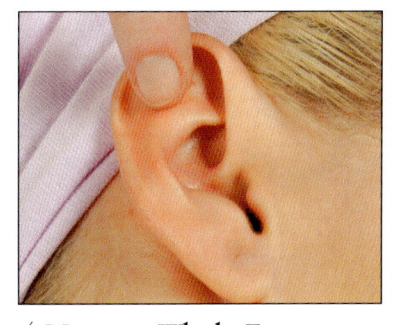

4 Massage Whole Ear

Massage the whole ear between your thumb and index finger, working from the lobes to the top of the ear.

Massage behind the ear, sweeping your index or middle finger up and down behind the ear lobe 2 or 3 times. Run your finger around the entire ear twice and finish by pulling on the lobes 3 or 4 times.

Return your hands to the starting position described on page 56 and gently massage the scalp to complete the sequence.

SIMPLY REFLEXOLOGY · 63

About the Author

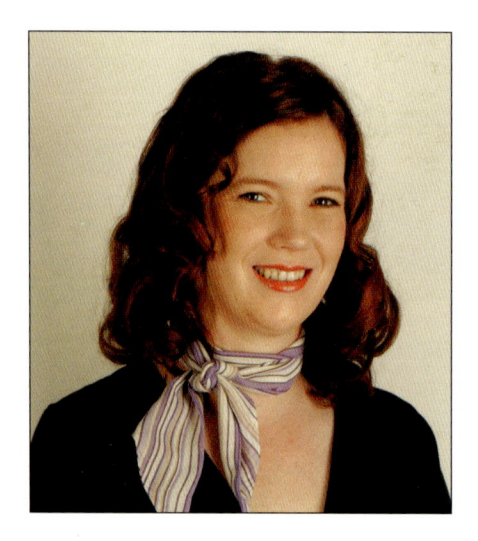

Claire Wynn is a fully qualified reflexologist and Swedish massage therapist. She has a holistic approach to healing and works with the client to promote and enhance their body's own natural healing ability. She aims to promote physical and mental wellbeing.

Claire started her studies in Scotland at the Scottish School of Reflexology and continued in Australia, obtaining a Diploma in Reflexology and Certificate IV in Massage at the Australian College of Natural Medicine, Brisbane. She also has a Certificate in Counselling Skills.

Claire currently has a clinic in Maleny, south east Queensland.